Igniting Your Liquid Intelligence

Integrating Modern Neurotransmitter Science with Ancient Ayurveda for Extraordinary Results

Robert Keith Wallace, PhD, Ted Wallace, MS, Carol Paredes, MS

Igniting Your Liquid Intelligence

ISBN 978-1-7357401-9-5

Library of Congress Control Number 2024921721

DharmaPublications.com

Dharma Publications, Fairfield, IA

To Our Very Dear Children and Grandchildren

OTHER BOOKS

Neurohacking for Online Learning
Study and Life Habits Optimized for Your
Personal Mind-Body Energy State
Robert Keith Wallace, PhD, Carol Paredes, MS

16 Super Biohacks for Longevity
Shortcuts to a Healthier, Happier, Longer Life
Robert Keith Wallace, PhD, Ted Wallace, MS, Samantha Wallace

Living in Balance with Maharishi AyurVeda
Practical Therapies for Consciousness-Based Health
Robert Keith Wallace, PhD, Karin Pirc, MD, Julia Clarke, MS

Self Empower
Using Self Coaching, Neuroadaptability, and Ayurveda
Robert Keith Wallace, PhD, Samantha Wallace, Ted Wallace, MS

Trouble in Paradise
How to Deal with People Who Push Your Buttons:
Using Total Brain Coaching
Robert Keith Wallace, PhD, Samantha Wallace, Ted Wallace, MS

The Coherence Code
How to Maximize Your Performance and Success in Business
For Individuals, Teams, and Organizations
Robert Keith Wallace, PhD, Ted Wallace, MS, Samantha Wallace

Total Brain Coaching
A Holistic System of Effective Habit Change
For the Individual, Team, and Organization
Ted Wallace, MS, Robert Keith Wallace, PhD, Samantha Wallace

The Rest and Repair Diet
Heal Your Gut, Improve Your Physical and Mental Health,
and Lose Weight
Robert Keith Wallace, PhD, Samantha Wallace,
Andrew Stenberg, MA, Jim Davis, DO, and Alexis Farley

Gut Crisis
How Diet, Probiotics, and Friendly Bacteria
Help You Lose Weight and Heal Your Body and Mind
Robert Keith Wallace, PhD, Samantha Wallace

Dharma Parenting
Understand Your Child's Brilliant Brain
for Greater Happiness, Health, Success, and Fulfillment
Robert Keith Wallace, PhD, Frederick Travis, PhD

Quantum Golf
The Path to Golf Mastery, REVISED Second Edition
Kjell Enhager, Robert Keith Wallace, PhD, Samantha Wallace

An Introduction to Transcendental Meditation
Improve Your Brain Functioning, Create Ideal Health,
and Gain Enlightenment Naturally, Easily, Effortlessly
Robert Keith Wallace, PhD, Lincoln Akin Norton

Transcendental Meditation
A Scientist's Journey to Happiness, Health, and Peace
Robert Keith Wallace, PhD

The Neurophysiology of Enlightenment
How the Transcendental Meditation and TM-Sidhi Program
Transform the Functioning of the Human Body
Robert Keith Wallace, PhD

Maharishi AyurVeda and Vedic Technology
Creating Ideal Health for the Individual and World
Robert Keith Wallace, PhD

The Coherence Effect
Tapping into the Laws of Nature that Govern Health,
Happiness, and Higher Brain Functioning
Robert Keith Wallace, PhD, Jay B. Marcus, Christopher S. Clark, MD

NOTE TO READER

Total Brain Coaching was originally published in 2019, introducing a comprehensive system for fostering effective change at the individual, team, and organizational levels. This foundational concept was further developed in three subsequent books: *Self Empower, 16 Super Biohacks for Longevity*, and *Neurohacking for Online Learning*. With this current book being the fifth in the series, we've dubbed it Total Brain Coaching 5.0. Alongside these core texts, we've also published companion works like *The Coherence Code* and *Trouble in Paradise*, which illustrate these principles through engaging fictional narratives. To date, thousands have benefited from courses inspired by the Total Brain Coaching system, reporting transformative results.

In 2023, a major leap forward was made in collaboration with a group of distinguished experts: Dr. Tony Nader, MD, PhD, one of the world's leading authorities in neuroscience and consciousness and author of the New York Times best-selling book *Consciousness Is All There Is;* Miriam Lodge, a top business consultant and consciousness expert; and Heather Evans, a renowned executive coach. Together, we developed the *SuperHabits* program that's been highly effective in driving personal and professional growth. We strongly recommend exploring this program further at superhabits.com.

This book offers a fresh perspective on self-development, focusing on how to optimize the "liquid intelligence" of your brain—the dynamic blend of neurotransmitters that shapes your thoughts, behaviors, and actions. We hope you find the journey enlightening and transformative. Enjoy!

CONTENTS

Introduction 1

Part I The Brain

    Chapter 1   Neuroplasticity in the Brain. 7

    Chapter 2   The Power of Brain Neurotransmitters. 13

    Chapter 3   Neural Circuits. 21

    Chapter 4   Dopamine Desire Circuit 29

    Chapter 5   Dopamine Reward Circuit 35

    Chapter 6   Here and Now Neurotransmitters. 41

    Chapter 7   Addiction 47

    Chapter 8   Stress and Dopamine Depletion 55

Part II Ayurveda

    Chapter 9   Basics of Ayurveda. 67

    Chapter 10 Understanding Vata. 77

    Chapter 11 Understanding Pitta 85

    Chapter 12 Understanding Kapha. 95

    Chapter 13 Daily Routine 103

    Chapter 14 Seasonal Routine 111

    Chapter 15 Ojas and Soma 119

Part III Strategies

    Chapter 16 Habit Change 127

    Chapter 17 Morning Sunlight 133

    Chapter 18 Diet and Digestion. 141

    Chapter 19 Gut Microbiome. 149

    Chapter 20 Supplements 157

    Chapter 21 Detox 165

Chapter 22 Sleep. 171

Chapter 23 Exercise 179

Chapter 24 Hydration and Cold Therapy. 187

Chapter 25 Breathwork 197

Chapter 26 Yoga Asanas 205

Chapter 27 Meditation 213

Chapter 28 Happiness 221

Chapter 29 Social Interactions. 229

Chapter 30 Spirituality 239

Chapter 31 Collective Consciousness 247

Part IV Appendices

Appendix 1 Energy State Characteristics 257

Appendix 2 Ayurvedic Diet and Digestion 271

Appendix 3 Transcendental Meditation. 281

Appendix 4 Group Dynamics of Consciousness. 289

References 295

About the Authors 329

Acknowledgments 331

Index. 333

INTRODUCTION

Tyler, a 33-year-old technical product executive coach, could be considered an overachiever. He finished college before he completed high school, taking night classes while his classmates were out partying. He landed his first corporate job at 14 and quickly rose to prominence as a top-tier executive coach by the age of 20. Known for his charisma, sharp insights into corporate dynamics, and remarkable results, Tyler's life was a whirlwind of travel, back-to-back meetings, coaching sessions, and speaking engagements. On the surface, he had it all—success, recognition, and a comfortable lifestyle. But beneath this polished exterior, unresolved issues simmered. His relentless drive for more—more success, more recognition, more achievement—was fueled by dopamine, the brain's motivator molecule. The constant rush of dopamine hits from conquering bigger challenges became the essence of his life. Yet, as Tyler's ambition climbed, so did his stress.

Then came the sudden disruption of the COVID-19 pandemic. Tyler's fast-paced life screeched to a halt. The frequent travel, constant challenges, and relentless dopamine surges he relied on abruptly stopped. Stress became a constant companion, and without his usual outlets, he turned to alcohol for relief. As a seasoned beer brewer who had won awards, Tyler initially saw drinking as just another competition—a contest he always intended to win. But alcohol soon hijacked his brain's reward system, replacing his once productive dopamine-driven career with an unhealthy dependency.

The consequences were severe. Alcohol's artificial stimulation of dopamine temporarily lifted Tyler's mood, but his brain adapted. He needed more alcohol to achieve the same effect, a classic sign of addiction. His baseline dopamine levels dropped, leaving him feeling flat and unmotivated when sober. The downward spiral infiltrated every part of his life, eventually leading to divorce and estrangement from his family.

> **At rock bottom—alone, exhausted, and physically deteriorating—Tyler realized he needed to change. His once powerful drive, which had fueled professional success, now threatened to destroy him.**

But Tyler's story wasn't over. He was able to use his inherent dopamine mechanism to publish two books, finding motivation again in writing. He then discovered running, initially to fill the void left by alcohol, but soon as a new source of dopamine-driven fulfillment. Starting with 10Ks and progressing to marathons, Tyler joined the "Marathon Maniacs," running marathons almost every other week. The exhilaration of improving his race times and finishing marathons began to replace the fleeting highs of alcohol.

Driven by his relentless ambition, Tyler didn't stop there—he trained for ultra-marathons, completing a grueling 100-mile race and even running a marathon in Antarctica. Running wasn't just a physical challenge; it became a means of rebalancing his brain, rechanneling his dopamine drive into something life-affirming. By leveraging the same neurochemical pathways that had once fueled his addiction, Tyler found healing, resilience, and a renewed sense of purpose.

Tyler's transformation is a microcosm of a broader crisis facing modern society. In today's fast-paced world, the combination of constant pressure and dopamine burnout is not just an individual problem; it has become a societal disruption. Stress and dopamine imbalances drive addiction, anxiety, burnout, and depression on a large scale. The need to understand and manage dopamine's role in motivation, reward, and resilience is more urgent than ever.

Decades earlier, Hans Selye, the pioneering endocrinologist, introduced the concept of stress as a biological response. His theory of the General Adaptation Syndrome (GAS) outlined three stages of stress adaptation: alarm, resistance, and exhaustion. While Selye's work focused primarily on hormonal stress responses, it laid the groundwork for understanding how stress affects the entire body, including the brain's dopamine pathways. Dopamine, as Selye didn't fully grasp in his era, is central to both the body's and the brain's response to stress. It plays a crucial role in the initial motivation to act, collaborating with other neurotransmitters to maintain function during resistance, but faltering during chronic stress—leading to burnout, reduced motivation, and even mental disorders.

During my own career, I (Keith) had the privilege of meeting Hans Selye in 1972 at a symposium held at Queens College, Canada, where Maharishi Mahesh Yogi, the founder of the Transcendental Meditation program, was the featured speaker. It was an extraordinary convergence of ancient wisdom and modern science, with Selye's ideas about stress adaptation blending intriguingly with Maharishi's teachings on consciousness and meditation. Maharishi proposed that meditation could not only reduce stress but also enhance well-being—an idea that aligns with our current understanding of how meditation affects neurotransmitter balance, particularly dopamine.

Maharishi was instrumental in bringing the ancient system of Ayurveda to the West, emphasizing its focus on balance and harmony within the mind and body. Ayurveda's principles resonate with modern neuroscience's findings about stress and dopamine management. Meditation, a core Ayurvedic practice, has been shown to regulate dopamine levels, enhancing feelings of reward and reducing stress. This balance mirrors the resistance phase in Selye's stress model, fostering mental resilience and adaptability.

> **The title, *Igniting Your Liquid Intelligence*, reflects the book's core message: to harness the fluid, dynamic nature of the brain's neurochemistry to foster mental adaptability and well-being.**

Dopamine, along with other neurotransmitters, constitutes a significant part of this "liquid intelligence"—the brain's ability to respond, adapt, and evolve. By understanding and optimizing the brain's dopamine pathways, we can unlock a new level of neuroadaptability, creating a perfect "brain cocktail" that supports resilience, creativity, and long-term health.

As we journey through this book, we'll delve into the science and practical strategies for optimizing brain function. We'll learn how to create the right mix of neurotransmitters to ignite our internal intelligence, enabling us to not only thrive in today's high-stress environment but also to lead more balanced, fulfilling lives. Through stories like Tyler's—and with the guidance of both modern neuroscience and ancient Ayurveda—we'll explore how to transform stress into strength, burnout into breakthrough, and liquid intelligence into lasting well-being.

PART I

The Brain

IGNITING YOUR LIQUID INTELLIGENCE

CHAPTER 1

NEUROPLASTICITY
IN THE BRAIN

The human brain is often compared to a supercomputer, but it is far more dynamic and adaptable. Neurons, the basic building blocks of the brain, communicate through a complex system of synapses—tiny gaps between nerve cells where neurotransmitters relay signals. This intricate electrochemical process allows neurons to "talk" to each other, awakening thought processes, generating emotions, and commanding physical movements.

At any given moment, your brain is teeming with activity, processing sensory input, making decisions, and navigating a complex landscape of emotions. To manage this complexity, the brain relies on key circuits—specialized pathways of neurons responsible for distinct functions such as memory, reward, stress response, and motor control. These neural circuits are powered by neurotransmitters, which are the liquid intelligence of the brain. When these circuits function harmoniously, mental clarity, emotional stability, and physical coordination follow. However, when imbalances occur, they can lead to mood disorders, cognitive impairments, or physical issues.

Jessica, a 35-year-old graphic designer, experienced the detrimental effects of such imbalances firsthand. Once celebrated for her creativity and meticulous attention to detail, she found herself mired in brain fog and low motivation after a particularly stressful year filled with demanding projects and tight deadlines. Simple tasks that had once been second nature now became sources of frustration, leaving her feeling stuck, not just in her work but also in her personal growth. The vibrant ideas that once flowed effortlessly felt trapped, overshadowed by an overwhelming sense of inertia.

Neuroplasticity: The Brain's Capacity for Change

> **One of the brain's most remarkable abilities is its capacity to change, adapt, and reorganize itself—known as neuroplasticity.**

Neuroplasticity refers to the brain's ability to form new connections between neurons, strengthen existing ones, or even create entirely new neural pathways in response to learning, experience, and environmental changes. This remarkable feature allows us to adapt to new challenges, recover from injuries, and learn new skills throughout our lives.

During childhood and adolescence, neuroplasticity is at its peak. The brain rapidly forms new connections as it absorbs information and experiences. This heightened plasticity is crucial for learning and development, allowing children to master language, social skills, and motor functions. However, as we enter adulthood, neuroplasticity becomes more selective, often leading to the pruning of unused synapses while reinforcing the most efficient pathways. This pruning process, essential for refining our abilities, can make the formation of new habits or learning complex skills more challenging.

Jessica discovered this selectivity when she decided to reclaim her creativity through new experiences. The constant stress had dulled her reward circuits, which thrived on creative break-throughs and achievements. Thanks to neuroplasticity, her brain could heal and adapt if she engaged in activities that stimulated those neural pathways.

Dopamine's Role in Neuroplasticity

Dopamine plays a critical role in neuroplasticity, acting as a key driver of the brain's ability to learn, adapt, and form new connections. This neurotransmitter is deeply involved in reward-based learning, motivation, and the reinforcement of new behaviors— all essential components of neuroplasticity.

When you learn something new or achieve a goal, dopamine is released in the brain's reward system, signaling success and encouraging repetition of the behavior. This surge in dopamine strengthens the connections between neurons involved in the learning process, making it easier for the brain to retain new information and repeat successful actions.

Jessica was determined to restore her creative spark by harnessing the power of dopamine. She began her journey with three key strategies aimed at enhancing her brain's neuroplasticity and boosting dopamine levels.

Learning a New Skill

Jessica decided to learn the piano, an instrument she had always admired but never had the chance to explore. At first, her fingers stumbled over the keys, and the notes sounded clumsy and dissonant. Yet, as she practiced and managed to play simple melodies correctly, she felt a rush of joy—each small success releasing dopamine and activating her reward circuits. This positive feedback loop not only improved her piano skills but also reignited her passion for creativity in other areas of her life.

Managing Stress Through Meditation

Recognizing that chronic stress had been a significant barrier to her creativity, Jessica committed to learning Transcendental Meditation (TM) and practicing it for twenty minutes twice a day. This practice not only helped restore her dopamine balance but also enabled her to approach work challenges with a clearer, more adaptive mindset. By managing her stress, she actively boosted her brain's capacity for change, ensuring that her dopamine levels were no longer depleted by constant tension.

Optimizing Lifestyle

Jessica also made lifestyle adjustments to support her brain health. Understanding the importance of sleep in consolidating new connections, she prioritized a consistent sleep schedule. She incorporated regular exercise into her routine, recognizing that physical activity could significantly increase dopamine release and improve overall brain function. Additionally, she revamped her diet, focusing on brain-healthy foods rich in omega-3s, antioxidants, and essential nutrients known to support neurotransmitter function.

The Balance of Stress and Neuroplasticity

While moderate levels of stress can enhance neuroplasticity by increasing dopamine release, chronic stress—like what Jessica had faced—depletes dopamine reserves, impairing the brain's ability to form new connections.

> **This is why managing stress is essential for maintaining cognitive flexibility and long-term brain health.**

After several months of commitment to her new practices, Jessica noticed remarkable improvements. Her creativity began to flow more freely, her motivation surged, and her work performance improved significantly. The vibrant ideas that had once felt trapped inside her began to resurface, and she rediscovered her love for graphic design. By actively engaging with neuroplasticity and optimizing her dopamine function, she transformed her mental landscape, regaining not just her professional edge but also a renewed sense of possibility in life.

Jessica's journey is a powerful testament to the brain's adaptability. Her experience illustrates that, regardless of the challenges we face, there is potential for growth and transformation. By understanding and harnessing the principles of neuroplasticity and dopamine optimization, anyone can unlock their full mental and physical potential, reclaiming their creativity and drive even in the face of adversity.

CHAPTER 2

THE POWER OF BRAIN NEUROTRANSMITTERS

Understanding neurotransmitters is essential to understanding how the brain works and how to optimize it for mental and physical health. More that 200 neurotransmitters have been identified, each having a different effect depending on the target cells they act on. Some can be excitatory, meaning they enhance the flow of information from one nerve to another, while others can be inhibitory, meaning they prevent the flow of information.

Neurotransmitters generally act after being released by one neuron and then flowing across the tiny synaptic gap between the two nerve cells and fitting into a receptor on the surface of a second neuron, like a key fitting into a lock. Once the neurotransmitter binds to the receptor, a chain of events is set in motion for a limited period of time. The neurotransmitter is then released from the receptor and either destroyed, or taken back up into the first neuron.

Different neurotransmitters have different effects, depending on where they act in the brain and what receptors they bind to. Let's take a closer look at some of the most critical neurotransmitters and how they shape your brain's performance.

Dopamine: The Motivator Molecule

Dopamine is primarily associated with reward, motivation, anticipation, and learning.

> **Dopamine plays a key role in goal-directed behavior, driving you to pursue activities that lead to rewards.**

When you achieve a goal—whether it's completing a task, reaching a milestone, or experiencing something pleasurable—dopamine surges, reinforcing the behavior and encouraging you to repeat it. Dopamine also regulates mood, energy levels, and voluntary movement. Imbalances in dopamine can contribute to various conditions, such as Parkinson's disease (due to dopamine deficiency in motor circuits) and addiction (due to overactivity in reward circuits).

Epinephrine and Norepinephrine: The Alert Molecules

Epinephrine and norepinephrine are also called adrenaline and noradrenaline and in addition to their role in awareness and attention they help to regulate many parts of the body such as blood pressure, heart rate, breath rate, and digestion. Epinephrine is mainly produced as a hormone from the adrenal glands and helps orchestrate the "fight or flight" response. Norepinephrine can act as a hormone, but primarily acts a neurotransmitter in the brain and sympathetic nerve endings. Its affects are generally slower and longer lasting than epinephrine.

Serotonin: The Mood Stabilizer

Serotonin is often referred to as the "mood stabilizer" because of its role in maintaining emotional balance and promoting feelings of well-being and happiness. It also regulates essential bodily functions, such as sleep, appetite, and digestion. Low levels of serotonin are strongly linked to depression, anxiety, and sleep disturbances. This is why many antidepressant medications work by increasing serotonin activity in the brain. Beyond mood regulation, serotonin also plays a role in social behavior and decision-making, particularly in contexts that require emotional regulation and impulse control.

GABA (Gamma-Aminobutyric Acid): The Brain's Brake System

GABA is the brain's primary inhibitory neurotransmitter, responsible for reducing neuronal excitability and preventing overstimulation. It functions as the brain's natural brake system, slowing down neural activity when neurons are firing too rapidly. This calming effect is crucial for maintaining a sense of relaxation, emotional stability, and reducing stress. Low levels of GABA are associated with anxiety, stress, insomnia, and certain mood disorders. It is also important for promoting restful sleep and preventing the kind of overactivity that can lead to conditions like epilepsy.

Glutamate: The Spark of Learning and Memory

Glutamate serves as the brain's principal excitatory neurotransmitter, driving the activation of neurons and fostering essential communication between them. Its role is paramount in brain development, as well as in the processes of learning and memory, where it enhances the efficiency of neural signaling. At the heart of this lies synaptic plasticity—the brain's remarkable ability to adapt by strengthening or weakening synapses, a mechanism crucial for memory formation and cognitive growth. Yet, while glutamate is indispensable for these vital functions, an overabundance can prove harmful. Excessive glutamate can lead to excitotoxicity, a state of overexcitation that causes neuronal damage. This process is linked to neurodegenerative disorders such as Alzheimer's disease and epilepsy, highlighting the delicate balance required for optimal brain function.

Acetylcholine: The Cognitive Enhancer

Acetylcholine is involved in many cognitive functions, particularly attention, memory, and learning. It also plays a role in controlling voluntary muscle movements. Acetylcholine helps to facilitate communication between neurons involved in memory formation and retrieval. In the peripheral nervous system, it helps control muscles, which is why a deficiency in acetylcholine can lead to problems such as muscle weakness or cognitive decline, as seen in conditions like Alzheimer's disease.

The Two Categories of Neurotransmitters

Neurotransmitters can be broadly categorized into two types: those that drive future-oriented, goal-directed behaviors, and those that regulate present-moment contentment and immediate responses. Drawing from *The Molecule of More* by Daniel Lieberman and Michael Long, dopamine stands at the center of the first category, fueling our pursuit of future rewards, motivation, and ambition. In contrast, epinephrine and norepinephrine, which prepare the body for immediate action during stress, are more aligned with "Here-and-Now" neurotransmitters. These chemicals, along with GABA, serotonin, and acetylcholine, foster present-moment focus, relaxation, and well-being. Glutamate plays a role in both categories, as it facilitates learning and memory for future planning while also enhancing neural communication in the present. This classification helps simplify our understanding of neurotransmitter functions by illustrating the two forces that shape human behavior: the relentless drive for future achievement and the capacity to find contentment and readiness in the present moment.

Dopamine: The Drive for More

Dopamine is future-oriented and responsible for motivating us to seek out new experiences, and push beyond our current state.

Dopamine propels us forward, encouraging us to chase rewards, take risks, and engage in ambitious pursuits. Dopamine is often referred to as the molecule of desire—it is not the pleasure itself but the anticipation and drive to pursue pleasure and success. However, because dopamine is focused on the future, it rarely allows us to feel truly satisfied. Instead, it keeps us on the hedonic treadmill, where we are always chasing more. Dopamine's influence is particularly strong in activities that involve novelty, risk, and potential rewards. This is why activities like gambling, substance use, or even social media engagement can hijack dopamine circuits, leading to addictive behaviors. The endless quest for more—whether it's more wealth, status, or stimulation—can become problematic when the brain's reward system is overstimulated.

"Here-and-Now" Neurotransmitters: Stability and Contentment

In contrast, "Here-and-Now" neurotransmitters—such as serotonin, oxytocin, endorphins, and norepinephrine—are focused on the present moment.

These neurotransmitters help regulate mood, promote relaxation, foster social bonds, and allow us to experience satisfaction and fulfillment in our current situation.

Serotonin promotes emotional stability and well-being, allowing us to feel content with what we have, rather than constantly seeking more. Oxytocin (also considered a hormone) fosters social connection and bonding, encouraging feelings of trust, love, and intimacy. Endorphins are your body's natural pain killers. Norepinephrine activates alertness and is part of the fight or flight response.

These neurotransmitters allow us to find joy, peace, alertness, and fulfillment in everyday life. They help us appreciate the here and now, rather than being constantly focused on the future or external rewards.

The Balance Between Dopamine and "Here-and-Now" Neurotransmitters

For optimal brain health, it is essential to maintain a balance between dopamine and "Here-and-Now" neurotransmitters. Dopamine, while crucial for motivation and achievement, can lead to restlessness and dissatisfaction when overemphasized. On the other hand, focusing too much on serotonin and other "Here-and-Now" neurotransmitters can result in complacency or a lack of ambition.

The key to mental well-being lies in balancing the drive for more with the ability to appreciate what we already have. By fostering both dopamine-driven ambition and serotonin-based contentment, we can maintain mental equilibrium, avoid burnout, and lead more fulfilling lives.

By cultivating a balance between ambition and contentment, we can harness the power of neurotransmitters to achieve extraordinary mental and physical results.

CHAPTER 3

NEURAL CIRCUITS

Lisa, a 45-year-old high school teacher, was celebrated for her enthusiasm and dedication in the classroom. Her students thrived under her guidance, inspired by her passion for learning. However, in the past year, Lisa found herself grappling with fatigue, lapses in memory, and emotional volatility. Her once-vibrant spirit was overshadowed by exhaustion, forgetfulness, and unpredictable mood swings. The root of Lisa's struggles lay in imbalances within her brain's neural circuits, the intricate pathways that govern motivation, memory, and emotional regulation.

Neural circuits are the highways of the brain, consisting of clusters of neurons that communicate to perform specialized tasks. While neurotransmitters like dopamine and serotonin provide the fuel for these circuits, it's their intricate connections that translate chemical signals into behavior. In Lisa's case, key circuits affecting her well-being included the dopamine reward circuit, the memory circuit, and the emotional regulation circuit.

Key Structures in the Brain

In the diagram, we observe several key structures in the brain. The dopamine reward circuit is split into two components: the dopamine desire circuit and the dopamine control circuit. Both circuits originate from a small group of cells located in the ventral tegmental area. The dopamine desire circuit transmits dopamine to the nucleus accumbens, whereas the dopamine control circuit delivers dopamine to the prefrontal cortex. We will explore each of these pathways in detail in the following chapters. Additionally, the amygdala plays a central role in the emotional circuit, while the hippocampus is crucial to the memory circuit.

Reviving Motivation with the Dopamine Reward Circuit

At the core of Lisa's professional drive was her dopamine reward circuit. This dopamine reward circuit plays a vital role in motivation, pleasure, and the pursuit of goals.

However, chronic stress had taken a toll, leading to diminished dopamine signaling and a lack of responsiveness in her reward system. Lisa found it increasingly challenging to connect with her students or develop engaging lesson plans.

After consulting a specialized life coach, Lisa learned how to reactivate her dopamine reward circuit. She started setting small, achievable goals each week—tasks like crafting an interactive lesson or organizing a fun class activity. Each completed goal provided a surge of dopamine, reinvigorating her motivation. As she experienced the rewarding feeling of accomplishment, her enthusiasm for teaching was reignited. This strategy not only helped her regain her passion but also fostered a sense of purpose that had been missing in her life.

Enhancing Memory through the Memory Circuit

Memory lapses became a source of frustration for Lisa, who often forgot student names or missed important deadlines. The coach explained that her memory circuit, centered in the hippocampus, was critical for encoding and retrieving information. This circuit heavily relies on neurotransmitters like acetylcholine and gluta-mate, which facilitate memory formation.

To strengthen her memory circuit, Lisa embarked on a jour-ney of mental engagement. She began learning a new language, an activity that required her to actively recall vocabulary and grammar rules. This exercise stimulated her hippocampus, pro-moting synaptic connections through increased acetylcholine and glutamate activity. Alongside her language studies, Lisa adjusted her diet, incorporating brain-healthy foods rich in choline and omega-3 fatty acids. Over time, her memory improved not only in her language lessons but also in her everyday teaching tasks. The renewed ability to recall names and details revitalized her confidence and effectiveness in the classroom.

Balancing Emotions with the Emotional Regulation Circuit

Lisa's most pressing challenge was her emotional landscape. Stress had exacerbated her feelings of irritability and sadness, and the coach shed light on the emotional regulation circuit that links the amygdala with the prefrontal cortex. The amygdala processes emo-tional reactions, while the prefrontal cortex helps regulate these responses. When stress levels rise, the amygdala can over-power the prefrontal cortex, leading to emotional dysregulation.

To restore balance, Lisa focused on boosting serotonin, a key neurotransmitter in emotional regulation. She began a daily gratitude journal, noting positive experiences and moments of joy. This simple practice enhanced serotonin activity, promoting emotional stability and empowering her prefrontal cortex to manage her emotional responses more effectively. Lisa also incorporated deep breathing techniques to calm her amygdala during stressful situations. As her emotional regulation circuit strengthened, she became less reactive and more composed, even in challenging classroom environments.

Managing Stress through the Stress Circuit

Lisa's stress response was governed by the hypothalamic-pituitary-adrenal (HPA) axis, a crucial component of the brain's stress circuit. Prolonged exposure to stress had resulted in an overactive HPA axis, leading to elevated levels of cortisol and adrenaline. These hormonal fluctuations contributed to her fatigue and emotional turmoil.

> **To moderate her stress response, the coach recommended a combination of aerobic exercise and the practice of Transcendental Meditation.**

Lisa dedicated 30 minutes each day to physical activity, discovering that this not only released dopamine and endorphins but also helped regulate her stress circuit. Additionally, she began practicing meditation for twenty minutes before and after work, which reduced cortisol spikes and increased her resilience to daily stressors. These changes not only enhanced her physical health but also contributed to a more balanced emotional state.

The Results: Balance and Well-Being

Over time, Lisa experienced a remarkable transformation. Her motivation surged, her memory improved, and she managed her emotions with newfound ease. By understanding and adjusting her neural circuits, she regained a sense of mental clarity and physical vitality. Lisa learned that while neurotransmitters fuel the brain, it is the circuits they operate within that ultimately dictate behavior.

Lisa's journey highlights the significance of recognizing and managing neural circuits to create positive changes in thoughts, behaviors, and emotions. By balancing the dopamine reward, memory, emotional regulation, and stress circuits, she not only revived her passion for teaching but also cultivated a sustainable sense of well-being.

The Importance of Neural Circuits

To fully grasp how the brain generates thoughts, emotions, and behaviors, we must delve deeper into the neural circuits that govern these processes. These circuits—such as the dopamine reward circuit, the memory circuit, and the emotional regulation circuit—are essential for mental and physical health.

The Dopamine Reward Circuit
This circuit is pivotal for motivation and pleasure-seeking behavior.

It involves projections from midbrain dopamine neurons to areas like the striatum and prefrontal cortex. When functioning optimally, it drives individuals toward rewarding activities and reinforces positive behaviors. However, chronic stress and other factors can impair this circuit, leading to decreased motivation and feelings of emptiness.

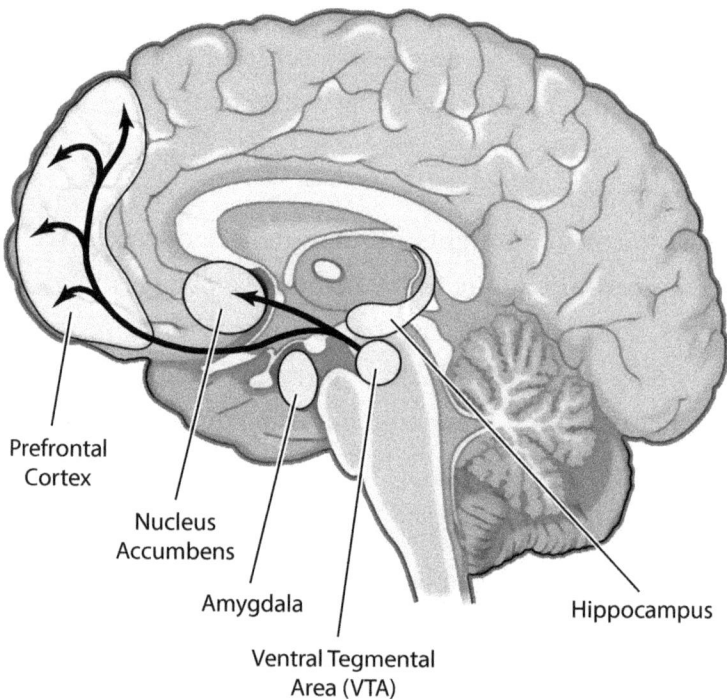

Cross-Section of the Human Brain

The Memory Circuit

Centered around the hippocampus, this circuit is crucial for encoding and retrieving experiences. Acetylcholine and glutamate are essential neurotransmitters in this circuit, promoting learning and memory. When disrupted, cognitive processes can falter, leading to memory issues and difficulties in learning.

The Emotional Regulation Circuit

This circuit connects the amygdala and prefrontal cortex, controlling how we respond to emotions. Serotonin plays a critical role in stabilizing mood and mitigating emotional reactivity. A healthy balance within this circuit enables individuals to manage stress effectively and respond to challenges with resilience.

The Stress Circuit

Governed by the HPA axis, the stress circuit prepares the body to respond to threats. Understanding how to manage this circuit is key to reducing stress-related symptoms and promoting overall well-being.

Conclusion: The Key to Well-Being

> **Maintaining balance within these neural circuits is vital for optimal brain function and overall health.**

By understanding how neurotransmitters influence these circuits, we can develop strategies to enhance our mental and emotional well-being. Lisa's journey illustrates the power of navigating the brain's highways—by optimizing her neural circuits, she not only revitalized her career as a teacher but also fostered a deeper sense of fulfillment in her personal life. In the upcoming chapters, we will explore the two main divisions of the dopamine reward system: the dopamine desire circuit and the dopamine control circuit.

CHAPTER 4

THE DOPAMINE DESIRE CIRCUIT

Ryan, a 32-year-old musician and entrepreneur, had always felt a deep passion for music. His days were filled with creative brainstorming, romantic pursuits, and ambitious business ventures, driven by a force he couldn't quite name. He was constantly inspired by new ideas, romantic feelings, and exciting goals. What Ryan didn't realize was that his boundless energy was fueled by the dopamine desire circuit—a neural network that drives anticipation, exploration, and forward-thinking.

Ryan thrived on imagining new possibilities. He spent countless hours in his studio, composing melodies and dreaming up ways to grow his small record label. The surge of dopamine in his brain made him feel unstoppable, pushing him to pursue both creative and romantic endeavors with enthusiasm.

However, Ryan's life wasn't without its challenges. While his desire for more propelled him toward new achievements, it also left him feeling restless and dissatisfied with the present moment. Let's explore how the dopamine desire circuit shaped different aspects of his life.

Creativity: The Spark of Innovation

Ryan's creative process was fueled by dopamine's anticipation-driven nature. He often described his songwriting sessions as "moments of flow," where ideas seemed to pour out effortlessly. The initial excitement of a new song concept came from the release of dopamine in his ventral tegmental area (VTA) and prefrontal cortex, enhancing cognitive flexibility and divergent thinking.

Yet, Ryan's creativity wasn't just about bursts of inspiration. The dopamine desire circuit also sustained his motivation to refine his compositions. Even when faced with a creative block, he remained driven by the anticipation of finishing a song. Each breakthrough—whether it was finding the right chord progression or finalizing lyrics—brought a dopamine rush that reinforced his desire to keep creating.

Ryan discovered that the secret to maintaining his creativity lay in setting both short-term and long-term goals. By breaking down big projects into manageable steps, he kept dopamine levels high throughout the process. This strategy allowed him to nurture his creativity without burning out, reinforcing his intrinsic motivation to explore new sounds and styles.

Love: The Chemistry of Connection

Ryan's love life was as intense as his creative pursuits. When he fell for someone, the dopamine desire circuit was fully activated, making him feel euphoric, focused, and eager to pursue the relationship. This sense of anticipation created feelings of excitement and joy, driven by increased dopamine activity in his VTA and nucleus accumbens.

In the early stages of his relationships, Ryan experienced what felt like "love at first sight," characterized by obsessive thinking, daydreaming, and a powerful urge to be close to his partner. The brain's anticipation of emotional intimacy, shared experiences, and future bonding fueled his desire to invest in the relationship. He often found himself taking risks and overcoming obstacles for love, driven by dopamine's motivating effects.

However, as the initial excitement faded, Ryan struggled with feelings of restlessness and dissatisfaction.

> **The dopamine desire circuit, wired to pursue new rewards, left him longing for novelty and fresh experiences even when things were going well.**

He realized that sustaining long-term love required balancing dopamine-fueled anticipation with serotonin-based contentment. By focusing on building deeper emotional bonds and shared goals, Ryan learned to maintain his romantic enthusiasm while finding fulfillment in the present.

For instance, he and his partner began to set time aside each week to discuss their dreams and aspirations, both personal and as a couple. This practice not only brought them closer emotionally, but it also fostered a sense of teamwork and shared purpose. Through these conversations, Ryan realized that the key to sustaining long-term passion was not just in grand gestures but in consistently nurturing the small, everyday moments that made their connection meaningful. Whether they were planning a future vacation together or simply enjoying a quiet evening at home, Ryan found joy in being fully present, knowing they were working towards a common future while appreciating the journey together.

Enthusiasm: The Engine of Engagement

Ryan's ambition wasn't limited to music and love—he was equally enthusiastic about growing his record label.

> **Every new business opportunity felt like an adventure, driven by the dopamine desire circuit's anticipation of success.**

Ryan often worked long hours, energized by the prospect of signing a new artist or launching a groundbreaking marketing campaign.

To sustain his enthusiasm, Ryan set clear milestones. For example, he celebrated signing a new artist or achieving a sales goal, which reinforced his motivation through incremental dopamine releases. Each achievement, no matter how small, felt like a step closer to his long-term vision. This approach kept him engaged and optimistic, even during challenging moments.

Ryan also found that dopamine's influence extended to how he handled setbacks. Rather than feeling discouraged, he reframed challenges as opportunities for growth, seeing them as part of the journey toward a bigger reward. This mindset, fueled by dopamine, allowed him to stay resilient and persistent, maintaining his enthusiasm through ups and downs.

The Blessing and Curse of Dopamine's Drive

While the dopamine desire circuit allowed Ryan to achieve

remarkable results in creativity, love, and business, it also had a dual nature. The constant focus on anticipation made it difficult for Ryan to feel satisfied with the present moment. He often found himself chasing the next big idea, the next romantic thrill, or the next business venture, unable to fully appreciate what he had already achieved.

Recognizing this, Ryan began integrating meditation into his daily routine. These practices helped him balance the desire for more with an appreciation for the present. By cultivating moments of stillness, he found greater contentment and maintained a healthier perspective on ambition and fulfillment.

The Key to Harnessing the Dopamine Desire Circuit

Ryan's story highlights the power and complexity of the dopamine desire circuit. It's a system that fuels creativity, passionate love, and enthusiasm, but also requires mindful management to avoid perpetual dissatisfaction. By understanding how dopamine drives anticipation and motivation, Ryan learned to channel his desires into meaningful, balanced experiences

CHAPTER 5

THE DOPAMINE CONTROL CIRCUIT

Ava, a 29-year-old marketing manager, was known for lighting up any room with her innovative projects and bold, out-of-the-box ideas. In the fast-paced world of digital marketing, her campaigns were nothing short of show-stopping. Driven by a thrill-seeking, dopamine-charged energy, she had an uncanny ability to spot trends, create buzz, and inject excitement into everything she touched. Yet, beneath her ambitious exterior lay a quieter struggle.

Though Ava could spark projects with boundless enthusiasm, she often found herself wrestling with the harder task of sustaining that fire. Weeks into her high-stakes campaigns, her initial momentum would wane, as new ideas sparkled on the horizon, luring her into starting yet another fresh, exciting project. This cycle—leaping from one idea to the next—highlighted an imbalance in her dopamine circuits: she thrived on the thrill of beginnings but faltered on the road to completion.

Realizing this, Ava began a journey to harness her ambition in a way that would let her see her visions through to the end. She sought ways to strengthen her self-discipline, to channel her energy so that her projects didn't just start with a bang but carried that excitement all the way to the finish line. It wasn't an easy path, but as she delved deeper into self-regulation, she discovered a new kind of thrill: the satisfaction that came from nurturing an idea from inception to impact. Little by little, Ava was learning not just to chase the dopamine highs of new beginnings but to find joy in the journey of seeing things through.

Struggling to Focus: Attention and the DLPFC

At work, Ava's bursts of creativity led to rapid productivity. Yet when tasks required sustained attention—like analyzing campaign data or preparing reports—her focus would drift. This struggle stemmed from a lack of dopamine activation in the dorsolateral prefrontal cortex (DLPFC), a key area responsible for executive functions such as attention and planning.

To improve her focus, Ava adopted strategies like breaking tasks into smaller, manageable chunks and setting clear deadlines. These practices helped boost dopamine levels in the DLPFC, making it easier for her to concentrate and resist distractions.

Impulse Control: The Role of the Basal Ganglia

Ava's impulsive tendencies extended beyond her work life. She often acted spontaneously, whether by making unnecessary online purchases, indulging in junk food, or checking her phone during meetings. These impulsive behaviors were driven by dopamine signals in the basal ganglia, particularly the caudate nucleus and putamen, which help suppress automatic responses.

Recognizing this pattern, Ava began practicing meditation to improve her impulse control. She focused on acknowledging her urges as they arose and intentionally delaying her responses by taking deep breaths. This simple pause activated her basal ganglia, enhancing her self-control and helping her regulate impulsive behaviors over time.

Decision-Making: Balancing Desire and Control

Ava's decision-making process was another area where she faced challenges. While she was quick to make bold moves in marketing, she often regretted hasty decisions—such as investing in new strategies without adequate research or agreeing to unrealistic timelines.

> **The DLPFC plays a crucial role in evaluating potential risks and rewards, and Ava's difficulties in making thoughtful decisions stemmed from insufficient dopamine activation in this region.**

To counter this, she began using a decision-making framework: listing pros and cons for each option and considering both immediate and long-term consequences. This structured approach helped activate her control circuit, allowing her to make more deliberate decisions that aligned with her long-term goals.

ADHD and the Control Circuit

Ava's challenges with attention and impulsivity were indicative of attention-deficit/hyperactivity disorder (ADHD). She went to a specialist and received a diagnosis of ADHD, which high-lighted the dopamine deficiencies in her prefrontal cortex and basal ganglia.

With her diagnosis, Ava began medication to increase dopa-mine levels in her control circuit. This pharmacological support, combined with cognitive-behavioral therapy (CBT), significantly improved her focus, decision-making, and impulse regulation. As she strengthened her dopamine control circuit, Ava found herself better equipped to manage her behaviors and maintain discipline in her work and personal life.

Balancing Ambition and Control

Ava's journey was about more than just strengthening her dopa-mine control circuit; it was about finding harmony between her ambition and self-regulation. While the desire circuit fueled her creativity and drive, the control circuit enabled her to channel that energy into focused, disciplined action.

To sustain this balance, Ava implemented routines that sup-ported both circuits:

Morning Exercise: Ava started her day with a 30-minute work-out, boosting dopamine in both the DLPFC and basal ganglia. This routine enhanced her mood and motivation, preparing her for the day ahead.

Meditation Practice: Daily practice of Transcendental Medita-tion increased activity in her prefrontal cortex and improved her impulse control. The calmness from meditation helped balance the high energy of her desire circuit.

Clear Goals and Rewards: Ava set specific, achievable goals

with small rewards along the way. This approach provided consistent dopamine reinforcement, keeping her motivated and focused on her long-term objectives.

Over time, Ava's efforts paid off. She experienced significant improvements in her ability to focus, regulate impulses, and make thoughtful decisions. By strengthening her dopamine control circuit, Ava achieved her goals with greater consistency and less stress. She learned that while ambition is a powerful motivator, it requires discipline and regulation to create lasting success.

The Anatomy of the Dopamine Control Circuit

> **The dopamine control circuit, which includes the DLPFC and basal ganglia, plays a critical role in maintaining self-discipline, attention, impulse regulation, and decision-making.**

This circuit works alongside the dopamine desire circuit to balance motivation with self-control.

Dorsolateral Prefrontal Cortex (DLPFC)

The DLPFC is essential for executive functions such as planning and decision-making. It regulates attention and helps maintain focus on tasks requiring sustained effort. By delaying gratification, the DLPFC empowers individuals to prioritize long-term rewards over immediate pleasures.

Basal Ganglia

The basal ganglia, located deep within the brain, are crucial for motor control, habit formation, and voluntary action regulation. Dopamine signals in the basal ganglia help suppress impulsive behaviors and prioritize actions that align with long-term objectives.

How the Dopamine Control Circuit Works

The dopamine control circuit regulates attention and manages impulses, focusing on inhibition rather than the pursuit of pleasure. It helps maintain focus on important tasks and reinforces goal-directed behavior through dopamine release in the DLPFC. By filtering out distractions and enabling self-control, the control circuit ensures that actions are aligned with long-term goals, fostering discipline critical for personal and professional success.

Ava's journey illustrates the importance of understanding and managing the interplay between the dopamine desire and control circuits. By strengthening her self-regulation and channeling her ambition, she discovered that true success lies not just in the pursuit of more, but in the balance between desire and discipline.

CHAPTER 6

HERE AND NOW
NEUROTRANSMITTERS

Mia, a 38-year-old software developer, was driven by an insatiable desire for more—more success, more experiences, more future achievements. This dopamine-driven ambition fueled her career, leading her to the upper echelons of her field, where she had everything from prestigious projects to lucrative bonuses. Yet with every milestone conquered, a familiar, hollow ache lingered, leaving her feeling perpetually restless and somehow...incomplete.

The thrill of her achievements dulled quickly, slipping away as her eyes set hungrily on the next target. Soon, her days felt like a blur of meetings and emails, and her nights turned into battles with racing thoughts and sleeplessness. She'd sit awake, scrolling mindlessly through social media, feeling trapped in an invisible cage of her own making, struggling to find any real sense of satisfaction. Her breakthrough came when she realized that no achievement could fill the void she felt inside.

After reaching out to a therapist, Mia was introduced to the concept of "Here and Now" (H&N) neurotransmitters. She learned that her constant drive for future rewards was fueled by dopamine but had come at the expense of other key neurotransmitters that foster present-moment joy: serotonin, oxytocin, and endorphins. These H&N neurotransmitters are the brain's way of grounding us in the moment, allowing us to feel genuine contentment, connection, and resilience.

> **The "Here and Now" neurotransmitters keep us present, enabling us to savor relationships, enjoy life's simple pleasures, and experience a deeper sense of fulfillment. While dopamine drives anticipation, H&N neurotransmitters help us appreciate what we already have.**

Serotonin: The Mood Stabilizer

Mia's therapist explained that serotonin, sometimes called the "feel-good" neurotransmitter, is crucial for stabilizing mood, promoting relaxation, and fostering a sense of contentment. Mia recognized that she rarely paused to celebrate her successes—always pushing herself toward the next big goal, perpetually striving and never feeling settled.

To boost serotonin, Mia began meditation and a daily gratitude practice. Each morning, after her TM practice, she listed three things she was grateful for on a whiteboard in her home office—simple joys like a warm cup of coffee or a sunny morning. Seeing these reminders throughout the day helped her stay connected to moments of joy, fueling her creativity, love, and enthusiasm, and allowing her to appreciate her present circumstances rather than constantly chasing more. This whiteboard habit also boosted her serotonin levels by maintaining a consistent focus on gratitude; each time she glanced at the board, her mind shifted from stress to appreciation, naturally increasing serotonin production in her brain. To further support her mood, Mia modified her diet to include foods like bananas, nuts, and dark chocolate, known for their serotonin-boosting properties. These small changes collectively helped Mia feel more grounded, stable, and increasingly content over time

Serotonin not only improves mood but also fosters present-moment awareness. It enables us to feel peace with where we are and what we have, reducing the urge to seek more. It plays a crucial role in regulating sleep, appetite, and digestion, making it vital for emotional stability.

Oxytocin: The Bonding Hormone

Ambitious at work, Mia often felt isolated in her personal life. As her therapist explained, this was partly due to a lack of oxytocin, the neurotransmitter responsible for emotional bonds and feelings of trust. Oxytocin fosters social connection, security, and intimacy, which are essential for well-being.

Mia decided to prioritize relationships by spending more time with loved ones. Simple acts like hugging, holding hands, or even petting her dog released oxytocin, deepening her sense of connection. She also practiced active listening, engaging fully in conversations without distractions. This shift allowed her to experience genuine intimacy, reducing her feelings of isolation and fostering emotional resilience.

Oxytocin not only enhances trust and bonding but also has a calming effect on the nervous system, reducing anxiety and promoting emotional regulation. It helps us feel connected to others, providing a sense of community and belonging that anchors us in the present.

Endorphins: The Natural Painkillers

While Mia's stress relief methods had often been dopamine-driven, like binge-watching TV or eating junk food, they provided only temporary satisfaction. Her therapist recommended more physical activities, which naturally release endorphins—neurotransmitters that help manage pain and elevate mood.

Mia started jogging three times a week. Initially, it was just a way to relieve stress, but she soon experienced the euphoric "runner's high," a result of the endorphin surge. This regular exercise made her feel not only happier but also more resilient, capable of handling both physical and emotional challenges. She also made a point of including more laughter in her life, whether through watching comedies or spending time with friends who made her laugh.

Endorphins play a vital role in managing stress and boosting emotional resilience. They help us experience joy even in the face of discomfort, allowing us to endure challenges while maintaining a positive outlook.

Balancing Dopamine with H&N Neurotransmitters

Mia's transformation wasn't just about increasing her H&N neurotransmitters—it was about balancing them with dopamine. Her ambition and drive were not inherently problematic, but they needed to be grounded by serotonin's calmness, oxytocin's connection, and endorphins' resilience.

To achieve this balance, Mia created routines that nurtured both dopamine and H&N neurotransmitters:

> Mindful Walks: Mia started taking daily walks without her phone, focusing on her surroundings. This practice combined present-moment awareness with a dopamine break, allowing serotonin to flourish.

> Connection Rituals: Mia established "no-phone dinners" with friends and family, enhancing oxytocin release through undistracted conversation.

> Exercise and Meditation: Mia alternated between jogging, walking, and meditation, integrating moments of endorphin highs with serotonin-driven stillness.

By integrating H&N neurotransmitters into her life, Mia no longer felt trapped in a constant pursuit of more. She found genuine joy in the present moment, with deepened relationships, improved mood, and a more stable sense of well-being.

Conclusion: The Importance of H&N Neurotransmitters

In modern society, we are often driven by dopamine—pursuing rewards, achieving goals, and seeking validation. While this drive can propel us forward, it can also lead to chronic dissatisfaction, anxiety, and burnout. The H&N neurotransmitters offer a vital counterbalance, allowing us to appreciate what we already have, foster meaningful connections, and experience true contentment.

Mia's journey illustrates how balancing dopamine with serotonin, oxytocin, and endorphins can lead to a more fulfilling life. By nurturing present-moment awareness and meaningful relationships, we can shift from a constant state of "wanting" to one of "being," experiencing a sense of peace, joy, and well-being that is both sustainable and deeply satisfying.

CHAPTER 7

ADDICTION

Gary, a 41-year-old construction worker, was once known for his laughter and easygoing spirit. He loved simple pleasures—barbecues with his family, Sunday softball games with friends, and the satisfaction of building things with his hands. But when a severe back injury struck, everything changed. Suddenly, the activities that once brought him joy became impossible, replaced by a daily battle with unrelenting pain.

His doctor prescribed opioids, and at first, the medication felt like a lifeline. It dulled the pain and allowed him brief moments of normalcy. But as the months passed, those brief moments became harder to reach. Gary found himself increasing the dosage, not just for relief but for an escape. The pills took the edge off his stress, replacing it with a fleeting, hazy euphoria—a temporary freedom from the reality of his limitations. He started relying on the medication to fill the emptiness he felt, telling himself it was only until he got back on his feet. But deep down, Gary sensed he was slipping. The man who once took pride in his strength and resilience was now haunted by a craving he couldn't quite control, feeling further and further from the life he used to love.

Gary's story exemplifies how addiction can hijack the dopamine reward circuit, transforming the brain's natural reward system into one focused solely on obtaining the addictive substance.

Dopamine Reward Circuit: A Brief Overview

The dopamine reward circuit is a neural network responsible for creating feelings of pleasure, motivation, and satisfaction. It helps us learn by reinforcing behaviors that lead to positive outcomes. The primary components of this circuit include:

- Ventral Tegmental Area (VTA): Where dopamine production begins, playing a central role in reward.

- Nucleus Accumbens: The area that generates feelings of pleasure and reinforces rewarding behaviors.

- Prefrontal Cortex: Governs self-control and decision-making.

Normally, this circuit encourages healthy, adaptive behaviors like eating, bonding, and achieving goals. However, addictive substances like opioids create unnaturally high levels of dopamine, hijacking this system and leading to compulsive behavior.

Gary's Descent: The Hijacking of Dopamine

Gary's addiction began as a physical necessity but soon spiraled into psychological dependence. Here's how his dopamine reward circuit was hijacked by addiction.

The Hijacking Begins: Dopamine Overload

Opioids provided Gary with an initial surge of dopamine in his VTA and nucleus accumbens, creating intense pleasure and relief.

> **This flood of dopamine signaled to Gary's brain that the drug was a highly valuable reward, reinforcing his desire to repeat the behavior.**

Over time, the brain adapted by reducing dopamine receptor availability—a process called receptor downregulation. This neuroadaptation made natural rewards, such as family time or hobbies, feel dull and less satisfying.

With repeated use, the euphoric effects diminished, prompting Gary to increase his dosage. His brain became reliant on opioids to feel pleasure, creating a vicious cycle of deeper dependency.

Neural Plasticity: Addiction's Grip

Gary's addiction wasn't just a chemical dependency; it became structural. The repeated use of opioids strengthened neural pathways that prioritized drug-seeking behaviors. As the reward circuit adapted, it began to override normal impulses, making the behavior habitual and automatic.

Gary's prefrontal cortex, responsible for self-control and decision-making, became impaired. Functional MRI studies show that addiction reduces prefrontal cortex activity, making it difficult to resist cravings. For Gary, this meant that even when he tried to stop using opioids, his brain's control circuit was too weakened to overcome the overpowering urges driven by the hijacked reward circuit.

Behavioral Consequences: The Cycle of Compulsion

Gary's addiction took a toll on every aspect of his life. He missed work, became distant from his loved ones, and struggled to maintain relationships. Despite his attempts to quit, intense cravings and withdrawal symptoms repeatedly drew him back to opioid use.

The dopamine control circuit, involving the dorsolateral pre-frontal cortex and basal ganglia, was too compromised to regulate his compulsive behavior. Gary's life became dominated by impulsivity and poor decision-making, preventing him from delaying gratification or resisting urges.

The Path to Recovery: Rewiring the Brain

Gary's turning point came after losing his job and facing legal troubles. Determined to change, he entered a comprehensive rehabilitation program that addressed both the neurochemical and behavioral aspects of addiction. His recovery involved several critical steps:

Medication-Assisted Treatment (MAT)
Gary was prescribed buprenorphine, a medication that partially activates opioid receptors without producing euphoria. This helped stabilize his cravings, restored dopamine balance, and reduced withdrawal symptoms, enabling Gary to focus on recovery.

Cognitive Behavioral Therapy (CBT)
CBT played a crucial role in Gary's recovery by helping him identify triggers and replace drug-seeking behaviors with healthier alternatives. This therapy strengthened his prefrontal cortex, improving impulse control and decision-making.

Exercise and Endorphin Boosts

Gary started exercising, which released endorphins—the body's natural painkillers. These endorphins alleviated his physical pain, elevated his mood, and gradually restored dopamine receptor sensitivity, making natural rewards more satisfying.

Transcendental Meditation (TM)

Gary also began practicing Transcendental Meditation, which research shows can enhance prefrontal cortex activity, reduce stress, improve self-control, and help eliminate addiction to a number of substances. TM helped Gary manage cravings and strengthened his dopamine control circuit, aiding long-term recovery.

Social Support and Connection

Gary joined a support group, finding camaraderie and understanding among others who faced similar struggles. This social bond released oxytocin, which reduced feelings of isolation and reinforced a sense of belonging that countered the loneliness of addiction.

Neuroplasticity and Long-Term Recovery

Over time, Gary experienced the benefits of neuroplasticity.

> **As he embraced new behaviors, his brain's reward system gradually became more sensitive to natural rewards like family time, physical exercise, and social connection.**

The neural pathways that once prioritized drug-seeking weakened, while new circuits supporting healthier habits and goals grew stronger.

Gary's recovery wasn't linear; he faced relapses, but each one offered insights into the triggers and neural mechanisms that fueled his addiction. By understanding how dopamine circuits had been hijacked and how they could be reshaped, Gary adapted his strategies, making gradual progress toward a more stable life.

The Complexity of Addiction

Addiction represents a powerful hijacking of the brain's dopamine circuits, making it a deeply challenging condition to overcome. However, as Gary's story illustrates, recovery is possible. By addressing the chemical, structural, and psychological aspects of addiction, individuals can regain control of their lives.

Treatment Approaches: Restoring Balance

Effective addiction treatment involves a multifaceted approach:

- Medication-Assisted Treatment (MAT): Stabilizes dopamine levels and reduces cravings.

- Cognitive Behavioral Therapy (CBT): Strengthens the control circuit and helps manage triggers.

- Exercise: Boosts endorphins and dopamine receptor sensitivity.

- Meditation (e.g., Transcendental Meditation): Enhances prefrontal cortex function, reducing stress and improving emotional regulation.

Support Groups: Build oxytocin-driven bonds that reduce isolation and provide accountability.

Conclusion: Finding Balance in Recovery

Gary's journey illustrates how addiction hijacks the dopamine reward circuit but also shows the brain's capacity for change. With targeted interventions and consistent effort, individuals can restore balance to their dopamine system and rebuild a fulfilling, addiction-free life.

Understanding the mechanisms of addiction and the role of dopamine can empower individuals to take control of their recovery. As seen in Gary's story, neuroplasticity enables the brain to adapt to new, healthier habits—replacing destructive cycles with pathways that lead to genuine well-being.

CHAPTER 8

STRESS AND
DOPAMINE DEPLETION

Emma, a 36-year-old emergency room nurse, thrived on the adrenaline-fueled energy of her job. Her passion for helping others and the fast-paced ER environment kept her going, with each high-stakes moment delivering a surge of dopamine that sharpened her focus and boosted her resilience. But as the years passed, the constant pressure started to weigh on her. What had once been an invigorating rush transformed into an exhausting routine. The unrelenting demands drained her dopamine reserves, leaving her feeling burnt out and disconnected from the sense of purpose that had once driven her.

Emma's journey reveals the often-overlooked link between chronic stress and dopamine depletion. As dopamine levels decline, the body struggles to find motivation and joy, creating a cycle that impacts both mental and physical health. Through Emma's experience, we see how long-term stress not only leads to burnout but also underlines the importance of addressing mental wellness in high-stress professions to preserve the balance that sustains motivation and well-being.

Dopamine and the Initial Stress Response

In the early days of her career, Emma thrived on stress. Each critical case triggered a dopamine surge from her ventral tegmental area (VTA) to her prefrontal cortex, heightening her focus, sharpening decision-making, and driving goal-directed behavior. Dopamine reinforced her motivation and rewarded her for effective crisis management, making each successful outcome feel like a small victory.

This phase was marked by high levels of adaptation, as dopamine helped Emma maintain alertness, energy, and goal-directed behavior. Her brain's reward circuit kept her engaged, ensuring she had the stamina to face even the most demanding situations.

Chronic Stress: Depleting Dopamine Reserves

However, as years of unrelenting stress accumulated, Emma's dopamine system became overtaxed. The initial surges of dopamine, which had once sharpened her performance, began to dwindle as her body struggled to sustain prolonged activation. The transition from acute to chronic stress brought several symptoms of dopamine depletion:

Loss of Motivation: Emma found it increasingly difficult to feel driven, even for tasks she had once enjoyed.

Emotional Numbing: The pleasure she once derived from hobbies, friendships, and even professional successes faded.

Cognitive Fatigue: Quick decision-making became a struggle, and mental clarity declined.

With chronic stress came prolonged cortisol exposure, further interfering with dopamine synthesis and receptor sensitivity. As dopamine signaling weakened, Emma's prefrontal cortex became less effective, impairing impulse control, decision-making, and emotional regulation. Symptoms of burnout—emotional exhaustion, depersonalization, and reduced personal accomplishment—set in.

Dopamine Burnout

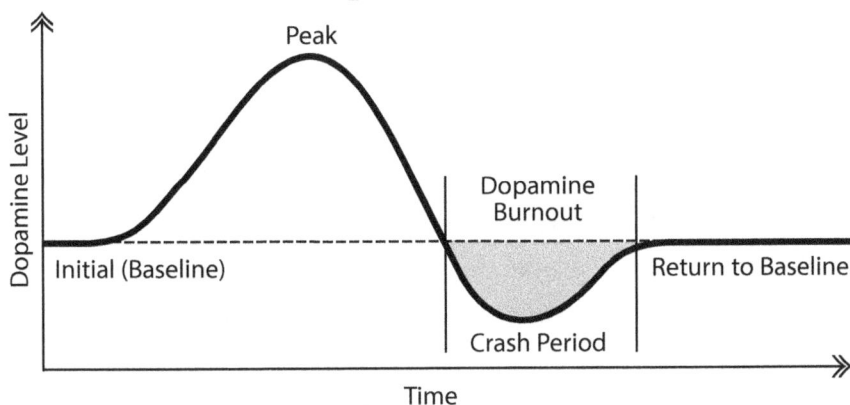

Restoring Balance: The Role of H&N Neurotransmitters

> **Emma's path to recovery began by focusing on H&N neurotransmitters, which play crucial roles in managing stress and aiding recovery.**

Engaging Oxytocin through Social Connections
During burnout, Emma's social life had taken a backseat. As part of her recovery, she made an effort to reconnect with friends, sharing her struggles openly. These interactions increased oxytocin,

promoting feelings of connection and support. Emma learned that seeking help was not a sign of weakness but an essential aspect of healing.

Calming with GABA

Emma struggled with insomnia, often lying awake replaying stressful events from work. To promote relaxation and restore her GABA levels, Emma practiced breathing exercises and took a warm bath before bed. This helped calm her mind, improve her sleep, and enhance her recovery from stress.

Enhancing Cognitive Flexibility with Acetylcholine

Emma began engaging in activities that challenged her cognitively, like puzzles and learning piano. These activities stimulated acetylcholine production, supporting mental flexibility, adaptability, and resilience—essential skills for managing high-stress situations.

Adaptability with Transcendental Meditation (TM)

Emma incorporated Transcendental Meditation into her daily routine, which helped lower cortisol levels and calm her overactive stress response. TM not only improved Emma's emotional regulation but also restored balance to her dopamine and serotonin systems, making her feel more connected to positive experiences.

The Impact of Chronic Stress: Burnout and PTSD

Emma's prolonged stress put her at risk for not only burnout but also Post-Traumatic Stress Disorder (PTSD). Heightened cortisol levels, combined with dopamine depletion, had created emotional numbness, a hallmark symptom of both conditions. Emma's therapy sessions helped her process traumatic experiences from the ER, alleviating PTSD symptoms and restoring her capacity for joy and fulfillment.

Stress and Dopamine Depletion

Stress activates the brain's dopamine system, driving motivation and focus during challenging situations. But prolonged stress can lead to dopamine depletion, which diminishes motivation, emotional engagement, and cognitive function. Understanding this dynamic is crucial for preventing burnout and managing chronic stress effectively.

Dopamine's Role in Stress Activation

- Sharpens focus by activating the prefrontal cortex.
- Boosts problem-solving and decision-making capacity.
- Reinforces goal-directed behavior, driving individuals to persevere through challenges.

The Shift from Activation to Depletion

- When stress becomes chronic, the brain's ability to produce dopamine diminishes.

Prolonged stress reduces the activity of dopaminergic neurons, leading to lower dopamine release.

The brain reduces dopamine receptor sensitivity to protect against overstimulation, making it harder to feel pleasure.

Elevated cortisol disrupts dopamine synthesis and reuptake, exacerbating feelings of fatigue, helplessness, and emotional numbness.

Recovery from Dopamine Depletion

Addressing dopamine depletion requires a comprehensive approach:

Cognitive-Behavioral Therapy (CBT): Reduces cortisol levels, indirectly supporting dopamine function.

Exercise: Boosts dopamine production and receptor sensitivity while promoting neuroplasticity.

Meditation (e.g., Transcendental Meditation): Lowers stress, improves emotional regulation, and restores dopamine balance.

Healthy Diet and Sleep: Tyrosine-rich foods and adequate sleep support dopamine production and receptor recovery.

Emma's Path Forward: Finding Joy Again

Emma's journey demonstrates that recovery from dopamine depletion involves both restoring dopamine levels and strengthening H&N neurotransmitters. By integrating physical, emotional, and social strategies, she not only overcame burnout but also developed greater resilience against future stress.

To reclaim her mental sharpness, Emma took on activities that stretched her brain in new ways. These activities naturally boosted her acetylcholine levels, a neurotransmitter that plays a vital role in enhancing cognitive flexibility, adaptability, and resilience. With each melody she mastered and puzzle she completed, Emma felt her mind becoming sharper and more agile, equipping her with essential skills to navigate the pressures of her demanding career with renewed strength and clarity.

Seeking relief from the cycle of stress, Emma turned to Cognitive-Behavioral Therapy (CBT), a proven approach to managing negative thought patterns. Through CBT, she learned to reframe her automatic responses, transforming her inner dialogue from self-critical and stress-fueled to balanced and constructive. This mental shift reduced her cortisol levels—the stress hormone that had been wearing her down—and indirectly supported her dopamine recovery, helping her regain motivation and emotional resilience. With each session, Emma felt empowered, building a toolkit of strategies to tackle stress and protect her well-being.

Emma's years in the ER took a significant toll on her mental health, placing her at risk for both burnout and Post-Traumatic Stress Disorder (PTSD). The combination of high cortisol levels and depleted dopamine left her feeling emotionally numb—a telltale sign of both burnout and PTSD. She found herself struggling with memories that wouldn't fade: the echo of sirens, the sight of distraught families, and the exhaustion from being perpetually on alert. These experiences, once manageable, now haunted her.

Through therapy, Emma was able to revisit and process these difficult moments. Her therapist offered her strategies to gradually reclaim her sense of control. Slowly, the numbness lifted, and with it, the intense weight of PTSD symptoms. With each session, Emma rediscovered her capacity for joy, reconnecting with the purpose that first drew her to the ER and restoring a newfound sense of fulfillment.

> **Emma understands that recovery isn't just about resting—it's about engaging in activities that restore her mental and emotional equilibrium.**

She schedules regular downtime to focus on activities that boost serotonin, GABA, oxytocin, and acetylcholine. Sunday mornings are reserved for a peaceful walk in the park, where the natural scenery lifts her mood and serotonin levels. Each morning and afternoon, she turns to yoga and Transcendental Meditation, to reduce anxiety and support relaxation.

To cultivate oxytocin, Emma makes time for cozy coffee dates with friends and snuggles with her beloved dog, reinforcing the connections that keep her grounded. And, to stimulate acetylcholine, she dedicates time to learning new piano pieces or solving puzzles, helping her stay mentally agile and engaged.

Emma is learning the power of setting small, meaningful goals that energize rather than exhaust her. She avoids overwhelming herself with ambitious targets and instead breaks her goals down into manageable steps. For instance, rather than aiming to master the piano all at once, she focuses on learning one piece each month. This approach provides regular dopamine boosts, reinforcing her motivation while keeping her efforts sustainable. Each achievement, no matter how small, serves as a positive milestone, keeping her spirits high without tipping into burnout.

Recognizing the importance of social bonds in managing

stress, Emma actively nurtures her relationships. She makes it a priority to connect with friends and family, whether through a shared meal, a heartfelt conversation, or a lighthearted video call. She also joins a support group for healthcare workers, where she can openly share her experiences with others who understand the pressures of her field. These moments of connection elevate her oxytocin levels, helping to buffer the impact of stress and providing a vital sense of community and resilience.

With a deeper awareness of her neurochemistry, Emma now approaches her work with renewed passion while maintaining balance. By nurturing dopamine and H&N neurotransmitters, she reclaimed her motivation, emotional stability, and cognitive flexibility.

IGNITING YOUR LIQUID INTELLIGENCE

PART II

AYURVEDA

CHAPTER 9

BASICS OF AYURVEDA

Ayurveda, the ancient system of health and wellness originating from India over 5,000 years ago, offers a holistic framework for understanding the mind, body, and spirit. It emphasizes balance—both internally within the body and externally with the environment. Central to Ayurveda's teachings are the doshas—the three fundamental energies that govern physiological and psychological functions. These doshas are known as Vata, Pitta, and Kapha. In this chapter, we will introduce these core Ayurvedic concepts and explore how they connect with modern understandings of neurotransmitters.

One of the goals of this exploration is to bridge ancient wisdom with modern neuroscience, especially by drawing parallels between the doshas and specific neurotransmitters. Before diving deeper into these connections, it is essential to first understand the foundational concepts of Ayurveda, particularly the doshas, Agni (digestive fire), and Ama (toxins). These core ideas shape how Ayurveda views health, disease, and balance.

The Doshas: Vata, Pitta, and Kapha

The doshas are the governing principles in Ayurveda that represent different combinations of the five elements (earth, water, fire, air, and ether) and control various physiological and psychological processes in the body. Every individual has a unique balance of these doshas, known as their prakriti (constitution), which dictates physical traits, mental tendencies, and overall health. While we will explore each dosha in greater depth in future chapters, a brief overview of their key characteristics is essential here.

Vata

Composed of air and ether, Vata governs movement, communication, and the nervous system. It is responsible for actions such as breathing, circulation, and neural transmission. People with a predominant Vata constitution are often creative, energetic, and quick-thinking, but when imbalanced, they may experience anxiety, insomnia, or digestive issues.

Pitta

Made up of fire and water, Pitta is linked to metabolism, digestion, and transformation. It governs body heat, digestion, and cognitive functions like intellect and focus. Balanced Pitta results in good digestion and sharp intellect, but excess Pitta can lead to anger, inflammation, or digestive disorders.

Kapha

Comprised of earth and water, Kapha provides structure, stability, and lubrication in the body. It is responsible for maintaining tissue health, strength, and emotional calm. People with a dominant Kapha dosha tend to be grounded, calm, and compassionate, but when Kapha is imbalanced, it can lead to lethargy, weight gain, and attachment to routine.

> **These doshas are not static; they constantly fluctuate in response to environmental changes, diet, lifestyle, and stress.**

Ayurveda teaches that maintaining harmony among the doshas is the key to health, and imbalances lead to disease.

Agni: The Digestive Fire

In Ayurveda, Agni is the concept of the "digestive fire" that governs all metabolic processes in the body. Agni is responsible for the digestion of food, absorption of nutrients, and the transformation of physical and mental energy. A strong Agni ensures optimal health, clarity of mind, and vitality, while a weakened Agni leads to the accumulation of toxins (Ama), disease, and mental fog.

From a modern perspective, Agni may be compared to metabolic processes and enzymatic functions, particularly those related to digestion and the nervous system's ability to metabolize information and stimuli. A balanced Agni supports mental sharpness and emotional stability.

Ama: The Source of Disease

Ama, in Ayurvedic terms, refers to undigested, toxic waste that accumulates in the body when Agni is weak or impaired. Ama clogs the body's channels and tissues, leading to a range of physical and mental ailments. It is the root cause of disease in Ayurveda, and the goal of treatment is often to eliminate Ama and restore balance to the doshas and Agni.

Symptoms of Ama include:

- Digestive discomfort such as bloating, gas, or constipation.

- Lethargy and heaviness in the body or mind.

- Coated tongue and foul breath, especially in the morning.

- Mental confusion, lack of clarity, or a sense of being "stuck."

In modern scientific terms, Ama could be compared to the buildup of metabolic waste or toxins in the body, similar to Leaky Gut Syndrome in which toxins and undigested food leak into the bloodstream. Once in the bloodstream, Ama then creates the basis for disease in various parts of the body.

The presence of Ama in the mind can be seen as analogous to mental "toxins" like stress and anxiety, which can disrupt neurotransmitter function, leading to imbalances in dopamine, serotonin, and GABA.

Ayurvedic treatment for Ama typically involves detoxification practices, such as panchakarma (a series of cleansing therapies), dietary changes, herbal remedies, and lifestyle modifications designed to strengthen Agni and cleanse the system of toxins. These approaches help to restore clarity, energy, and balance by supporting both the digestive system and the mind.

Maharishi AyurVeda: A Modern Adaptation of Ancient Wisdom

Maharishi AyurVeda, developed by Maharishi Mahesh Yogi, integrates the timeless wisdom of Ayurveda with modern scientific research. It places a strong emphasis on the mind-body connection and the role of consciousness in health. One of the cornerstones of Maharishi Ayurveda is Transcendental Meditation (TM), a technique designed to reduce stress, balance the doshas, and restore harmony to the nervous system.

In Maharishi AyurVeda, TM is seen as essential for supporting Agni and eliminating Ama, as it helps the body recover from the effects of stress and promotes overall well-being. This practice is also thought to enhance the function of neurotransmitters to promote calmness and mental clarity.

Additionally, Maharishi AyurVeda advocates for personalized health plans that align with each individual's doshic constitution, considering their lifestyle, environment, and mental state. By combining traditional Ayurvedic approaches with modern research on the mind-body connection, Maharishi AyurVeda offers a comprehensive method for achieving health and wellness in the modern world.

A Bridge Between Ancient and Modern Understanding

Ayurveda provides an intricate and holistic view of health that remains profoundly relevant today.

The concepts of the doshas, Agni, and Ama form a foundation for understanding how the body and mind work in harmony, and how imbalances can lead to disease. As we continue to explore the connections between Ayurveda and modern neuroscience, we will see how the wisdom of ancient traditions can enhance our understanding of brain function and neurotransmitter balance.

A number of published scientific studies that have explored the scientific basis of Vata, Pitta, and Kapha. Studies have examined the correlation between Ayurveda and gene expression. In fact, a whole new field of study has emerged called Ayurgenomics which examines the relationship between the three dosha types and gene expression. The dosha types have also been correlated with specific systems in the brain. In one interesting paper Vata dosha is related specifically to dopamine.

In the following chapters we will examine our own theory of how both Vata and Pitta are related to dopaminergic circuits in the brain and how Kapha relates to the H&N neurotransmitters.

Who are You?

Ayurveda emphasizes staying balance. Why is it so easy for some people to stay in balance while for others it's hard? We are all different and the sooner we discover who we are, the sooner we can improve our lives. Ayurveda and many other systems of traditional health have a procedure for understanding what is best for each of us. They personalize health and learning.

Let's take a simple quiz to find out your dosha type according to Ayurveda. A far more complete approach would be to see a qualified Ayurvedic physician or Vaidya who would do a thorough examination that included a pulse evaluation. But this quiz will give you valuable insights into who you are and how you can stay in balance. We describe the doshas in terms of Energy States of the body. Complete all three of the three quizzes shown below, rating yourself on a scale of 1 to 5, where 1 signifies "strongly disagree" and 5 represents "strongly agree".

Energy State Quiz

V (Vata) Energy State	Strongly Disagree — Agree				
1. Light sleeper, difficulty falling asleep	[1]	[2]	[3]	[4]	[5]
2. Irregular appetite	[1]	[2]	[3]	[4]	[5]
3. Learns quickly but forgets quickly	[1]	[2]	[3]	[4]	[5]
4. Easily becomes overstimulated	[1]	[2]	[3]	[4]	[5]
5. Does not tolerate cold weather very well	[1]	[2]	[3]	[4]	[5]
6. A sprinter rather than a marathoner	[1]	[2]	[3]	[4]	[5]
7. Speech is energetic, with frequent changes in topic	[1]	[2]	[3]	[4]	[5]
8. Anxious and worried when under stress	[1]	[2]	[3]	[4]	[5]
V Score	(Total your responses)				

P (Pitta) Energy State	Strongly Disagree — Agree				
1. Easily be- comes overheated	[1]	[2]	[3]	[4]	[5]
2. Strong reaction when challenged	[1]	[2]	[3]	[4]	[5]
3. Uncomfortable when meals are delayed	[1]	[2]	[3]	[4]	[5]
4. Good at physical activity	[1]	[2]	[3]	[4]	[5]
5. Strong appetite	[1]	[2]	[3]	[4]	[5]
6. Good sleeper but may not need as much sleep as others	[1]	[2]	[3]	[4]	[5]
7. Clear and precise speech	[1]	[2]	[3]	[4]	[5]
8. Becomes irritable and/or angry under stress	[1]	[2]	[3]	[4]	[5]
P Score	(Total your responses)				

K (Kapha) Energy State	Strongly Disagree — Agree				
1. Slow eater	[1]	[2]	[3]	[4]	[5]
2. Falls asleep easily but wakes up slowly	[1]	[2]	[3]	[4]	[5]
3. Steady, sta-ble temperament	[1]	[2]	[3]	[4]	[5]
4. Doesn't mind waiting to eat	[1]	[2]	[3]	[4]	[5]
5. Slow to learn but rarely forgets	[1]	[2]	[3]	[4]	[5]
6. Good physical strength and stamina	[1]	[2]	[3]	[4]	[5]
7. Speech may be slow and thoughtful	[1]	[2]	[3]	[4]	[5]
8. Possessive and stubborn under stress	[1]	[2]	[3]	[4]	[5]
K Score	(Total your responses)				

Compare all three scores. Whichever total is higher, V, P, or K, is your primary Energy State. It is common to have two high scores and one lower score. This shows that you are a combination of two main Energy States, with a minor influence from the third. In some cases, you may have three similar scores. This is somewhat rare and indicates that you are a Tri-Dosha or Tri-Energy State.

CHAPTER 10

UNDERSTANDING VATA

Meet Leah, a 34-year-old painter whose life vividly embodies the essence of the Vata dosha. Her world is one of boundless creativity, quick-thinking insights, and a contagious enthusiasm that lights up every room she enters. Ideas seem to flow through her effortlessly, and she's always on the hunt for fresh inspiration—whether in her art or her next adventure. This lively pursuit of the new mirrors Vata's mobile, light, and spontaneous qualities, reflecting a natural harmony with the dopamine-driven desire for novelty and excitement.

Leah's story beautifully illustrates the synergy between the Vata dosha and our brain's dopamine desire circuit. While this energetic force fuels her originality and zest for life, it also reveals the potential challenges of Vata: if unbalanced, her drive for change and stimulation can become overwhelming. This balance of Vata's gifts and its pitfalls invites us to explore ways to channel our energy while staying grounded, allowing us to embrace the beauty of Vata without being swept away by its currents.

The Spark of Vata: Creativity and Mobility

Leah's Vata nature was evident in her creative pursuits. As a painter, she constantly generated new concepts, experimenting with various artistic styles. This surge of creative energy was fueled by Vata's mobile, light, and quick-moving qualities, which correspond to the dopamine release in her ventral tegmental area (VTA) and nucleus accumbens. This dopamine activity sustained Leah's motivation, enabling her to explore fresh ideas and push creative boundaries.

> **Vata's movement is not only physical but also mental—fueling Leah's rapid thinking and curiosity.**

She often felt a dopamine-driven rush of excitement while envisioning new projects or anticipating professional recognition, perfectly reflecting Vata's forward-oriented nature.

Vata and Dopamine: The Drive for More

Leah's Vata energy extended beyond her creative work to her lifestyle. She loved trying new activities—whether learning to play the guitar, starting a fresh fitness routine, or planning spontaneous trips. This pursuit of novelty mirrored dopamine's role in stimulating goal-directed behavior and seeking new rewards.

However, Leah also struggled with the downside of Vata and dopamine's forward-looking nature. Her enthusiasm for "more" often left her feeling restless and unsatisfied. She had difficulty staying grounded, frequently jumping from one project to another without finishing them. Just as dopamine emphasizes anticipation over fulfillment, Vata thrives on the excitement of planning rather than experiencing the present moment.

The Downside: Vata Imbalance and Overactive Dopamine

As Leah's workload increased, her irregular routines and constant search for new stimuli began to overwhelm her system, resulting in classic Vata imbalances:

Anxiety: Leah's mind became overactive, filled with racing thoughts and urgency. This mental overstimulation reflected the excess activation of her dopamine desire circuit, driving her need for constant action and novelty.

Digestive Issues and Insomnia: Vata's cold, dry, and irregular qualities manifested physically in digestive issues, causing bloating and inconsistent appetite. Leah's racing mind made it difficult to wind down at night, leading to insomnia.

Emotional Exhaustion: Leah's relentless drive for new projects eventually led to emotional depletion, a sign of both dopamine depletion and excessive Vata. She felt empty and disconnected from the activities that once brought her joy.

The overstimulation of both Vata and the dopamine desire circuit can result in anxiety, burnout, and emotional numbness when left unchecked.

Finding Balance:
Grounding Vata and Replenishing Dopamine

Recognizing the need for balance, Leah turned to Ayurveda to calm her Vata energy while also addressing her dopamine-driven behavior. Here's how Leah restored equilibrium:

Grounding Practices
Leah adopted grounding activities to counteract Vata's light and mobile qualities:

▌ Warm baths and self-massage (abhyanga) with warm sesame oil promoted physical and mental stability.

▌ Regular meals with warm, moist foods, like soups and stews, helped regulate digestion and provided nourishment.

▌ Sipping hot water throughout the day.

▌ Maintaining a daily routine.

These practices anchored her energy, reducing the mental restlessness associated with both Vata and dopamine excess.

Meditation and Breathwork
Leah found relief through Transcendental Meditation (TM), which helped calm her racing thoughts and reduce anxiety. TM supported dopamine regulation by promoting present-moment awareness, counteracting Vata's tendency toward future-oriented thinking. She also incorporated slow, deep breathing (pranayama) to relax her nervous system and balance Vata.

Establishing Regular Routines
Leah set consistent wake-up and sleep times, which improved her sleep quality and stabilized her mental state. Although establishing routines was challenging, it was essential for managing Vata's irregularity.

Creative but Balanced Outlets
Leah continued engaging in creative projects but focused on fewer

at a time. She incorporated breaks for rest and reflection, ensuring her creativity remained a source of joy rather than a drain.

Nourishing Foods
Leah shifted her diet to include Vata-balancing foods that also support dopamine production, such as bananas, avocados, almonds, and cooked vegetables. This dietary change stabilized her digestion while maintaining her mental energy.

Social Connection for Emotional Support
Leah prioritized meaningful social interactions, increasing oxytocin and reducing feelings of isolation. This shift helped calm her overactive Vata energy while also reinforcing dopamine through positive social bonds.

Vata and Dopamine: Understanding the Connection

Vata is the dosha of movement, creativity, and mental activity, while dopamine is the neurotransmitter of motivation, reward, and novelty-seeking. Both drive action, exploration, and the pursuit of new experiences. Here's how they align.

Creativity and Novelty
Vata's imaginative qualities are closely linked to dopamine's role in promoting cognitive flexibility and a desire for novelty. Individuals with a dominant Vata dosha often possess an abundance of innovative ideas, similar to how elevated dopamine levels encourage divergent, creative thinking.

Restlessness and Anticipation
Both Vata and dopamine are future-oriented, focusing more on anticipation than present fulfillment. This tendency can lead to restlessness and dissatisfaction.

Motivation and Mental Movement
Vata's light and mobile nature fuels mental activity and goal-directed behavior, mirroring dopamine's role in stimulating reward-seeking pathways.

When Vata and Dopamine Become Imbalanced

While both Vata and dopamine are essential for creativity and motivation, imbalances can lead to physical and mental health issues:

Excessive Vata and Dopamine
Overstimulation results in restlessness, anxiety, impulsivity, and burnout. This parallels the mental and physical effects of excessive dopamine activity.

Deficient Vata and Dopamine
Lack of Vata movement leads to mental dullness and lethargy, akin to the effects of low dopamine, which reduce motivation and cognitive flexibility.

Strategies for Balancing Vata and Dopamine

Ayurveda offers strategies to restore balance:

Grounding Practices

Regular routines, gentle exercise, and warm, nourishing foods stabilize Vata and regulate dopamine.

Meditation

Practices like TM help calm Vata, support dopamine regulation, and promote present-moment awareness.

Herbs

Ayurvedic herbs like ashwagandha and brahmi reduce Vata imbalances and support nervous system health.

Balanced Stimulation

Engaging in creative endeavors while ensuring rest and recovery maintains Vata's dynamism without overstimulating dopamine pathways.

Leah's Path Forward: A Balanced Approach to Creativity

> **Leah's journey shows how balancing Vata and dopamine can lead to sustainable motivation and creativity.**

By understanding the interplay between Vata's qualities and dopamine's influence, Leah found a harmonious blend of inspiration, motivation, and calm. She learned to harness her creativity without falling into cycles of restlessness or burnout.

In today's fast-paced world, the constant drive for achievement can push Vata and dopamine systems into overdrive. By integrating Ayurvedic principles with insights from neuroscience, individuals can maintain a balance that fosters innovation, well-being, and peace.

CHAPTER 11

UNDERSTANDING PITTA

Raj is a 42-year-old financial analyst whose life is a testament to the essence of Pitta dosha. Sharp, disciplined, and purpose-driven, Raj's days are marked by intense focus and a commitment to excellence that make him stand out in his field. His knack for analytical precision and his ability to stay calm under pressure make him a natural in high-stakes environments, where others look to him for leadership and solutions. Raj's personality reflects Pitta's fiery, transformative qualities, mirroring the influence of the dopamine control circuit—a system in our brain that fuels focus, self-regulation, and the relentless pursuit of goals.

Raj's story showcases the powerful synergy between Pitta and the dopamine control circuit, illustrating how this alignment can drive remarkable success. But it also hints at the potential challenges of such intensity: when this energy becomes unbalanced, the same fire that fuels achievement can lead to burnout and stress. Raj's journey invites us to explore the strengths and vulnerabilities of Pitta, encouraging us to harness this energy for growth while finding ways to keep it balanced and sustainable.

Pitta's Fire: Focus and Transformation

Raj's Pitta nature was the driving force behind his career success. He thrived in intense situations, solving complex financial problems with ease and making strategic decisions quickly. Pitta's heat, sharpness, and intensity were evident in Raj's ability to maintain focus, prioritize tasks, and transform ideas into results.

> **The dopamine control circuit, especially in the dorsolateral prefrontal cortex (DLPFC), was key to Raj's success.**

Dopamine activity in this part of the brain enabled Raj to regulate impulses, maintain attention, and organize tasks effectively. Pitta's transformative energy aligned with the dopamine control circuit, allowing Raj to stay disciplined, sharp, and clear-headed under pressure.

Goal-Oriented Drive: Achieving Success

Raj is highly goal-oriented, setting clear objectives in both his professional and personal life. Whether completing a major financial report or achieving a fitness milestone, Raj's ability to break down complex tasks into manageable steps was a hallmark of both Pitta and the dopamine control circuit.

Raj's intense focus helped him sustain motivation over time, ensuring progress toward long-term goals. This drive, fueled by Pitta's transformative qualities and dopamine's structured regulation, made Raj successful in achieving tangible results.

The Downside: Overcontrol and Burnout

While Raj's Pitta energy and dopamine control circuit supported his disciplined nature, they also led to imbalances that impacted his mental and emotional well-being.

Perfectionism

Raj often set impossibly high standards for himself and others. His need for structure and precision, driven by an overactive dopamine control circuit, made him inflexible. He struggled to adapt when plans changed, leading to frustration and self-criticism.

Anger and Irritability

Pitta's heat manifested as frequent bouts of anger, especially when things didn't go as planned. Raj's rigid focus on achieving goals, combined with the dopamine control circuit's drive for order, made him prone to outbursts when expectations were not met.

Burnout

Raj's relentless pursuit of goals led to physical and mental exhaustion. Pitta's fiery energy, when not regulated, contributed to overexertion, while the dopamine control circuit's rigidity led to mental fatigue and difficulty balancing work demands with personal well-being.

Deficient Pitta: Lack of Focus and Motivation

Raj once faced a period of Pitta deficiency, brought on by prolonged stress and burnout. His characteristic sharpness and unwavering drive began to fade, leaving him struggling with focus and motivation. It was as if the fire that once fueled his ambitions had dwindled, reflecting an underactive dopamine control circuit—a system that typically supports focus, self-regulation, and goal-oriented energy. Raj's story highlights how the depletion of Pitta energy can disrupt our natural momentum, underscoring the importance of balance for sustained clarity and purpose.

Lack of Motivation
Without Pitta's usual intensity, Raj found it hard to stay focused on long-term goals, leading to procrastination and indecision. His weakened dopamine control circuit made it difficult to maintain momentum, leaving tasks unfinished.

Mental Fog
Raj's usual clarity was replaced by mental dullness. Simple decisions became overwhelming as dopamine activity declined, leaving Raj feeling lost and ungrounded.

Balancing Pitta and the Dopamine Control Circuit

To regain balance, Raj integrated Ayurvedic and neuroscience-based strategies that restored his mental sharpness, emotional stability, and overall well-being.

Cooling Practices
To reduce Pitta's heat, Raj adopted a cooling diet and lifestyle:

Cooling Foods
Raj incorporated cucumbers, leafy greens, coconut water, and other cooling foods into his diet to pacify Pitta.

Gentle Yoga and Evening Walks
These activities dissipated excess heat and soothed Raj's mind, tempering the intensity of both Pitta and the dopamine control circuit.

Meditation and Breathwork
Raj found relief through meditation, which calmed his mind and reduced overactivity in the dopamine control circuit. He also practiced deep, slow breathing (pranayama) to manage anger and promote relaxation. These techniques helped Raj maintain mental clarity without becoming overly rigid or frustrated.

Structured Routines with Flexibility
Raj maintained a structured routine but learned to incorporate breaks and downtime. He scheduled regular "off time" for rest, which allowed for spontaneity and adaptability. This approach helped prevent perfectionism and enabled Raj to adapt to unexpected changes without stress.

Regular Exercise
While Raj continued exercising, he chose less intense forms, like swimming and cycling, which reduced Pitta's intensity without

aggravating competitiveness. This balanced exercise routine helped regulate dopamine, supporting mental clarity and emotional well-being.

Herbal Support

Raj started taking Ayurvedic herbs, such as brahmi and shatavari, known for their cooling properties and ability to support cognitive function. These herbs helped maintain Pitta's clarity while reducing its heat.

Avoiding "Hangry" Moments

Raj discovered that irregular eating triggered irritability—a classic Pitta imbalance. He started eating small, frequent meals that were nutrient-dense and cooling, such as salads, lentils, and herbal teas. This strategy helped prevent dips in blood sugar, which can deplete dopamine and intensify Pitta's fiery nature.

Pitta and the Dopamine Control Circuit: Structure and Discipline

While Vata is linked to creativity and novelty through the dopamine desire circuit, Pitta aligns more closely with the dopamine control circuit, which governs self-regulation, focus, and impulse control. Here's how Pitta and the dopamine control circuit work together.

Focus and Attention

Pitta's mental sharpness corresponds to the dopamine control circuit's ability to sustain focus. When balanced, this connection supports clarity, planning, and decision-making.

Impulse Control and Discipline

Pitta's intensity helps maintain discipline, much like the dopamine control circuit's role in regulating impulses and maintaining order.

Goal-Oriented Behavior

Pitta's drive for results aligns with dopamine's function in maintaining focus on long-term goals, breaking complex tasks into manageable steps.

When Pitta and Dopamine Become Imbalanced

Imbalances in Pitta and the dopamine control circuit can lead to:

Excessive Pitta

Overcontrol, perfectionism, and anger. This parallels an overactive dopamine control circuit, where excessive focus can lead to rigidity and burnout.

Deficient Pitta

Lack of focus, motivation, and mental fog. This corresponds to an underactive dopamine control circuit, resulting in lethargy, indecision, and reduced clarity.

Strategies for Balancing Pitta and Dopamine

Ayurvedic practices can help regulate Pitta while supporting dopamine control.

Cooling Practices

Incorporate cooling foods and activities to prevent Pitta from overheating and to reduce rigidity in the dopamine control circuit.

Meditation

Helps calm the mind, reduce stress, and promote mental flexibility, counteracting both Pitta's intensity and dopamine's overcontrol tendencies.

Structured Flexibility

Maintaining routines with built-in downtime prevents Pitta from becoming overly rigid while supporting dopamine regulation.

Regular Nourishment

Eating regular, balanced meals helps stabilize blood sugar and prevent drops in dopamine, reducing irritability and mental fatigue.

Raj's Path Forward: A Balanced Approach to Focus

> **By integrating cooling, grounding, and restorative practices, Raj learned to harness his Pitta energy without becoming overwhelmed by intensity or perfectionism.**

He maintained his focus and drive while achieving a sense of inner calm and balance.

In a fast-paced world, it's easy for Pitta and the dopamine control circuit to become overactive. By combining Ayurvedic insights with neuroscience, individuals can create a balanced approach that fosters clarity, discipline, and well-being—without compromising emotional stability.

CHAPTER 12

UNDERSTANDING KAPHA

Maya is a 46-year-old elementary school teacher, whose life beautifully exemplifies the essence of Kapha dosha. Calm, patient, and nurturing, Maya has a quiet strength that creates a safe and consistent environment for her students and colleagues alike. Known for her steady, reassuring presence, she brings a sense of stability that those around her deeply appreciate. Her personality embodies the grounded qualities of Kapha, which provide physical strength, emotional resilience, and a deep sense of stability.

Maya's story illuminates the powerful connection between Kapha and the "Here-and-Now" neurotransmitters, which promote emotional well-being, social connection, and inner calm. Her Kapha nature supports her ability to live fully in the present, offering her students a sense of warmth and security that encourages them to thrive. Yet Maya's journey also reveals the potential pitfalls of excessive Kapha: when this dosha is imbalanced, the same qualities that make her so dependable can lead to stagnation, lethargy, or difficulty adapting to change. Maya's life reminds us of the beauty in Kapha's nurturing energy and the importance of balancing it to stay dynamic and energized.

Kapha's Strength: Stability and Connection

Maya's Kapha energy was evident in her physical build and emotional stability. She had a strong, well-built body, characteristic of Kapha's heavy and stable qualities.

> **Her calm demeanor exuded warmth and empathy, creating a nurturing environment for her students. Maya's grounded nature aligned with key H&N neurotransmitters.**

Serotonin

Maya's steady serotonin levels supported her calm and content demeanor, enhancing emotional stability, resilience, and well-being. Serotonin, like Kapha, fosters balance, helping Maya maintain her composure even during stressful situations.

GABA

Maya's natural relaxation and composure reflected balanced GABA levels, which act as a brake on neural excitability. GABA's calming effect aligned with Kapha's slow and steady nature, allowing Maya to remain patient and clear-headed, even in chaotic situations.

Oxytocin

Maya's nurturing presence was rooted in oxytocin, the neurotransmitter of bonding and trust. Her deep, lasting relationships mirrored Kapha's soft and compassionate qualities, creating a sense of safety and connection.

Excess Kapha: Stagnation and Emotional Heaviness

While Maya's Kapha energy brought emotional resilience and nurturing, it also led to imbalances.

Physical Stagnation

Over time, Maya noticed weight gain, sluggishness, and a lack of motivation to exercise. Her body's natural tendency toward heaviness, combined with a sedentary lifestyle, mirrored serotonin imbalances, often linked to feelings of lethargy and low mood.

Emotional Attachment

Maya found it hard to let go of past relationships and experiences. Excessive oxytocin, like excessive Kapha, can foster overattachment, making it difficult for her to move forward.

Depression

Maya experienced emotional heaviness and sadness, resembling low serotonin levels. Despite her usual contentment, she struggled to find joy in everyday activities.

Deficient Kapha: Anxiety and Instability

When Maya's school underwent major restructuring, she experienced a temporary deficiency in Kapha. The sudden changes disrupted her usual sense of stability.

Emotional Instability

Without Kapha's grounding energy, Maya felt anxious and

ungrounded, mirroring low GABA levels that contribute to anxiety and nervousness.

Social Disconnection

Maya, who normally thrived on connection, withdrew and felt isolated. This social withdrawal resembled low oxytocin levels, leading to feelings of loneliness and a loss of emotional support.

Balancing Kapha and H&N Neurotransmitters

> **To restore balance, Maya embraced Ayurvedic and neuroscience-based strategies to regain stability, calmness, and connection.**

Stimulating Movement

To counter physical sluggishness and boost serotonin levels, Maya began a morning walking routine and light exercise. This increased her energy, lifted her mood, and reduced feelings of heaviness.

Social Engagement

Maya made a conscious effort to reconnect with friends, enhancing oxytocin. She joined a community gardening group, which allowed her to nurture plants and bond with others—combining Kapha's nurturing qualities with oxytocin's bonding effects.

Meditation for Relaxation

Maya practiced deep breathing and meditation, which calmed her mind and enhanced GABA activity. This helped her maintain relaxation without slipping into stagnation, allowing her to remain calm and centered, even amidst change.

Nourishing, Balanced Diet
Maya adjusted her diet to include warm, light foods with bitter and astringent tastes, reducing Kapha's heaviness. She also added foods that support serotonin production, like eggs, and nuts, enhancing her mood and emotional resilience.

Flexible Routines
Maya introduced flexibility into her structured routines by trying new activities or spontaneously visiting friends. This prevented rigid patterns and kept her energy adaptable.

Kapha: The Principle of Stability

Kapha governs physical strength, emotional resilience, and groundedness. Composed of earth and water elements, it offers:

- Physical strength and endurance through heavy and steady qualities.

- Emotional stability and patience with its slow, cool, and nurturing nature.

- Steadiness in routines and relationships, providing continuity and security.

When Kapha is balanced, it fosters calmness, compassion, and long-lasting bonds. However, excess Kapha can lead to lethargy, depression, and attachment, while deficiency can result in anxiety and instability.

Kapha and H&N Neurotransmitters: The Power of Presence

Kapha's characteristics align with the H&N neurotransmitters:

- Serotonin: Supports mood stability and emotional resilience, reflecting Kapha's calming qualities.

- GABA: Promotes relaxation and quiets the mind, mirroring Kapha's stabilizing influence.

- Oxytocin: Fosters social bonding and connection, enhancing Kapha's nurturing presence.

These neurotransmitters help maintain calm and emotional stability, reinforcing Kapha's grounding energy.

When Kapha and H&N Neurotransmitters Become Imbalanced

Imbalances in Kapha and H&N neurotransmitters can lead to:

Excess Kapha
Physical and emotional stagnation, lethargy, and depression. Excessive serotonin can lead to emotional heaviness, while overattachment linked to oxytocin can result in clinging behavior.

Deficient Kapha
Anxiety, restlessness, and social disconnection. Low GABA levels can cause heightened nervousness, while low oxytocin can lead to

feelings of isolation.

Avoiding Emotional Stagnation and Attachment

Maya learned to avoid Kapha's tendency toward emotional attachment by staying open to change and new experiences. Engaging in stimulating activities, maintaining social bonds, and allowing for spontaneity helped Maya balance her nurturing qualities with adaptability.

Nurturing Kapha for Emotional Resilience

Maya's journey shows that Kapha's strength lies in its grounding, nurturing energy, which fosters emotional stability and resilience. By integrating movement, social connection, meditation, and a balanced diet, Maya maintained her natural strengths while avoiding stagnation and attachment.

> **In a world that often demands rapid change, balancing Kapha with H&N neurotransmitters offers a path to calm, contentment, and well-being.**

Through Ayurveda and neuroscience, we can nurture Kapha's enduring qualities while embracing flexibility and growth.

CHAPTER 13

DAILY ROUTINE

Rina, a 39-year-old sociology professor, found herself struggling with a sense of physical and mental instability. Her energy levels fluctuated, mood swings became more frequent, and an underlying feeling of imbalance started to seep into her work and personal life. Eager to regain a sense of control, Rina was intrigued by Ayurveda's personalized approach to wellness, particularly drawn to the concept of dinacharya, or the Ayurvedic daily routine, as a pathway to establish stability and harmony.

Rina's journey illustrates the transformative power of a daily routine tailored to her unique dosha. Through consistent practices that aligned with her natural rhythms, Rina not only regained her physical health but experienced a boost in neurotransmitter function, enhancing her mood, motivation, and emotional resilience. Her story reveals how a mindful, Ayurvedic routine can become a foundation for lasting well-being, bringing a sense of balance that radiates through every aspect of life.

Identifying Rina's Dosha: Vata Predominance

Rina's Ayurvedic practitioner identified her as predominantly Vata, characterized by lightness, movement, and irregularity.

Rina's quick, creative mind was fueled by Vata's qualities, but her scattered schedule and late-night work habits left her feeling ungrounded and mentally exhausted.

Her daily routine needed to balance Vata while also supporting neurotransmitters like dopamine, serotonin, GABA, and acetylcholine—all crucial for mental stability and focus.

Morning Routine: Waking Early to Stimulate Motivation

Rina started waking up at 5:30 AM, during the Brahma Muhurta, a time associated with mental clarity and Vata energy.

> **Initially, waking up early was tough, but soon she noticed significant improvements.**

Cortisol Regulation
Waking up aligned with her body's natural cortisol rise, making her feel more alert and energized. This cortisol boost helped initiate a steady rise in dopamine, increasing motivation and readiness for the day.

Sunlight Exposure
Stepping outside for morning sunlight helped regulate her circadian rhythm and suppress melatonin, promoting alertness. Sun exposure also increased serotonin levels, lifting her mood and stabilizing energy throughout the day.

Morning Rituals

Rina's morning rituals were designed to cleanse and energize her body.

Tongue Scraping and Warm Water

Each morning, Rina began her day with the practice of tongue scraping, using a specially designed metal or copper scraper. Tongue scraping is an Ayurvedic practice that involves gently removing the coating that can build up on the tongue overnight. This coating, which may contain bacteria, toxins, and residual food particles, is considered a form of Ama (toxic buildup) in Ayurveda. By removing it, tongue scraping helps to stimulate digestion and awaken the flow of Agni (digestive fire), preparing her digestive system for the day ahead.

Following tongue scraping, she would drink a glass of warm water to further support digestion. This simple yet powerful practice activates her metabolism and gently flushes the system, setting a foundation for balanced digestion throughout the day. Together, these practices became a morning ritual that revitalized her digestion and left her feeling refreshed and energized.

Gentle Yoga and Pranayama

She followed a 20-minute session of gentle yoga and breathing exercises, focusing on slow, grounding movements that balanced her Vata energy. This activated acetylcholine, improving mental clarity and enhancing focus for the workday.

The regularity of these rituals brought Rina newfound stability, allowing her to start each day with focus and calmness.

Meditation

Rina incorporated Transcendental Meditation (TM) for 20 minutes each morning, finding it to have profound effects on her mood.

Serotonin Boost

Regular meditation elevated serotonin levels, reducing anxiety and improving emotional stability. Rina felt more grounded, free from the restless thoughts that often plagued her Vata mind.

GABA Activation

Meditation's calming effects promoted GABA activity, reducing Rina's overstimulation. It helped her transition smoothly from rapid mental energy to a more stable, balanced state of mind.

Tailored Routine for Vata Balance

> **Rina's daily routine helped to balance her Vata tendencies.**

Regular Mealtimes

Rina established consistent mealtimes, ensuring warm, cooked meals with spices like ginger and cumin. This stabilized her digestion and prevented erratic energy dips. Regular meals maintained balanced dopamine levels, providing sustained motivation and focus.

Grounding Foods
Incorporating grounding foods like sweet potatoes, lentils, and avocados balanced Vata's lightness and dryness while supporting serotonin production, promoting a sense of contentment.

Gentle Evening Routine
A calming evening routine, including warm baths with lavender oil and light stretches, helped Rina unwind and prepare for restful sleep, further supporting GABA and serotonin balance.

The Impact on Neurotransmitters: Balanced Mood and Motivation

Rina experienced profound changes as she continued with her routine.

Improved Motivation
Early waking and sunlight exposure kept her dopamine levels steady, boosting motivation and focus. She was more productive and less prone to distractions.

Calmer Mood
Meditation and grounding foods stabilized serotonin, reducing anxiety and promoting a steady mood. Rina felt more emotionally resilient.

Better Relaxation
Regular breathing exercises, meditation, and a structured evening routine enhanced GABA levels, allowing for deeper relaxation and

improved sleep quality. Her mind felt clearer, and erratic thoughts that once kept her awake diminished.

Ayurveda's Daily Routine: Dinacharya and Neurotransmitters

> **Modern neuroscience aligns with Ayurveda in emphasizing the importance of routine. Regular habits help regulate the brain's neurotransmitters, creating stability and reducing stress.**

Dopamine
Structured routines support the dopamine system, enhancing motivation and focus.

Serotonin and GABA
Habits that promote calm, such as meditation or consistent mealtimes, boost serotonin and GABA, stabilizing mood and promoting relaxation.

Acetylcholine
Morning rituals and mental stimulation activate acetylcholine, improving focus and mental clarity.

Tailoring the Daily Routine for Vata, Pitta, and Kapha

Ayurveda recommends adjusting routines based on the dominant dosha.

Vata

Routines for Vata types should emphasize warmth, grounding, and regularity. Practices like gentle yoga, warm foods, and structured schedules help prevent anxiety and erratic energy.

Pitta

Pitta types benefit from routines that include cooling activities, regular breaks, and meditation to avoid burnout. Cooling foods and soothing evening routines help manage intensity and maintain balance.

Kapha

Kaphas need invigorating routines, with stimulating morning exercise, light meals, and engaging social interactions to prevent lethargy.

Rina's Takeaway: Routine as a Path to Well-being

Rina's journey highlights the power of dinacharya, showing how it can harmonize doshas and neurotransmitters. By integrating daily practices that align with Ayurvedic principles and the science of neurotransmitters, Rina achieved a sustainable balance in her physical health, mental clarity, and emotional stability.

The Ayurvedic daily routine offers a structured approach that optimizes neurotransmitter function, supporting well-being at all levels. Tailoring these routines to individual constitutions makes them more effective, helping maintain a harmonious blend of productivity and inner calm.

CHAPTER 14

SEASONAL ROUTINE

Arun, a 34-year-old AI expert, often found himself feeling off-balance as the seasons changed. Mood swings, shifts in energy, and occasional digestive upsets seemed to arise unpredictably, leaving him searching for solutions beyond his usual wellness habits. Intrigued, he consulted an Ayurvedic practitioner, who suggested that his struggles might be linked to seasonal influences on his doshas and recommended ritucharya—the Ayurvedic practice of adjusting one's routine with each season.

Following this advice, Arun began to incorporate small yet powerful changes into his daily life to reflect nature's rhythm. His meals, exercises, and sleep patterns were adjusted to honor each season's unique qualities, helping him align with the natural shifts in energy and neurotransmitter patterns throughout the year. As he embraced this seasonal approach, Arun noticed profound changes: his mood became steadier, his energy more consistent, and his digestion more resilient.

Arun's story reveals how Ayurvedic seasonal routines can harmonize our body's rhythms with the changing environment. By aligning with nature, we can cultivate balance, mental clarity, emotional stability, and a vibrant sense of well-being, season after season.

Arun's Ayurvedic Constitution: Vata-Pitta Dosha

Arun's constitution was identified as Vata-Pitta, with Vata's light, dry, and irregular qualities and Pitta's sharp, intense, and fiery traits. His Ayurvedic practitioner emphasized the need to tailor his routine according to the seasons to balance both Vata and Pitta while supporting key neurotransmitters like dopamine, serotonin, and GABA. Common to all seasons, Arun practiced morning and evening meditation for enhancing GABA and serotonin levels, calming the mind, and reducing irritability.

Arun learned how each season corresponds to a different dosha, influencing both his physical state and neurotransmitter balance:

Vata Season (Late Autumn to Early Winter): Cold, dry, and windy conditions are associated with dopamine fluctuations and serotonin instability.

Pitta Season (Summer): Heat and intensity can trigger dopamine overload and GABA dysregulation.

Kapha Season (Late Winter to Spring): Cool, damp, and heavy qualities can lead to serotonin drops and reduced motivation.

Vata Season

As late autumn approached, Arun noticed increased anxiety, restlessness, and dry skin—classic Vata imbalances. His practitioner suggested grounding and warming routines to balance Vata and stabilize neurotransmitter function.

Here's what Arun's Vata-season routine included:

Warm, Nourishing Foods

Arun added soups, stews, and root vegetables to his diet, helping him feel grounded and emotionally stable. The warm, cooked foods provided steady energy, supporting dopamine production and preventing mood swings.

Regular Routine

Arun set consistent times for waking, eating, and sleeping, which regulated serotonin levels and reduced anxiety.

Oiling the Body (Abhyanga)

Daily self-massage with warm sesame oil calmed the nervous system and promoted relaxation, reducing overstimulation and supporting GABA activity.

Gentle Exercise and Yoga

Arun chose slow, grounding exercises like yoga and Tai Chi to maintain circulation without overstimulating his nervous system, stabilizing dopamine and serotonin levels.

Consistent Sleep and Rest

Arun established a regular bedtime routine, improving sleep quality and maintaining balanced dopamine and serotonin levels.

Pitta Season

> **During the Pitta season, Arun felt irritable, impatient, and experienced occasional skin breakouts—signs of Pitta imbalance.**

Arun's practitioner recommended cooling strategies to manage Pitta and prevent neurotransmitter dysregulation. Arun's Pitta-season routine included:

Cooling Foods
Arun incorporated cucumbers, leafy greens, and coconut water into his diet, which not only reduced Pitta's heat but also stabilized serotonin levels, preventing emotional volatility.

Cooling Herbs
Adding mint, coriander, and fennel to meals helped maintain a calm mind and prevented dopamine overload.

Cooling Exercise
Arun focused on swimming and slow yoga during cooler parts of the day to maintain steady dopamine flow without overheating.

Avoiding Spicy Foods
Arun avoided hot, spicy foods that could further aggravate Pitta, opting instead for bitter and astringent tastes that cooled his system.

Kapha Season

As late winter transitioned into spring, Arun felt heavy, sluggish, and experienced low motivation—signs of Kapha imbalance.

> **His practitioner recommended invigorating practices to counter Kapha's heaviness and boost neurotransmitter function.**

Arun's Kapha-season routine included:

Light, Spicy Foods
Arun's meals were lighter and included warming spices like ginger, black pepper, and turmeric, which stimulated serotonin production and improved mood.

Vigorous Exercise
Unlike in Vata and Pitta seasons, Arun needed more vigorous exercise during Kapha season to boost dopamine and endorphins. Cardio, brisk walking, and strength training helped maintain energy and motivation.

Mental Stimulation
Arun engaged in activities like puzzles, learning new skills, and socializing to support dopamine production and prevent mental sluggishness.

Avoiding Dairy and Heavy Foods
Arun reduced dairy and heavy foods, which could increase Kapha's heaviness. Instead, he focused on lighter meals that maintained clarity and motivation.

Early Rising

Arun made an effort to wake up early, taking advantage of the lighter mornings to stimulate energy and mood, supporting serotonin and dopamine regulation.

Adapting to the Seasons: Neurotransmitter and Dosha Balance

By implementing ritucharya, Arun experienced significant improvements in his mood, energy, and overall well-being. Aligning his lifestyle with the changing seasons not only balanced his doshas but also stabilized neurotransmitter function, enhancing mental clarity and emotional resilience.

> Serotonin Stability: Warm foods in Vata season, cooling foods in Pitta season, and light meals in Kapha season helped maintain serotonin levels, promoting emotional stability and reducing mood swings.

> Dopamine Regulation: Seasonal exercise and dietary practices kept dopamine balanced, maintaining steady motivation and preventing burnout or lethargy.

> GABA Enhancement: Regular meditation, grounding activities in Vata season, and cooling practices in Pitta season supported GABA function, reducing stress and promoting relaxation.

The Key to Seasonal Adaptation

Arun discovered that ritucharya is not rigid but a flexible, adaptive approach to maintaining balance. By aligning his habits with seasonal changes, he found more resilience and joy in each phase of the year. Seasonal routines offered unique opportunities for growth, adaptation, and well-being.

In Ayurveda, the seasonal routine is foundational for maintaining harmony and health. It aligns the body's doshas and neurotransmitters with nature's rhythms, supporting both physical and mental well-being throughout the year. By understanding and adapting to these seasonal shifts, we can ensure that both the body and mind remain balanced, resilient, and vibrant year-round.

CHAPTER 15

OJAS AND SOMA

Tara, a 45-year-old holistic health coach, had dedicated much of her life to wellness, yet she couldn't shake a lingering feeling of depletion and a yearning for a deeper, more profound spiritual experience. Despite her commitment to health practices, she felt that something essential was missing. Inspired by Ayurveda's teachings on Ojas—the subtle energy of vitality—and Soma, the nectar of bliss, as described by Maharishi Mahesh Yogi in relation to higher states of consciousness, Tara began to explore these ancient concepts as pathways to enhance both her physical energy and spiritual depth.

Eager to nourish her Ojas and awaken the qualities of Soma, Tara immersed herself in practices that aligned her body, mind, and spirit. Through diet, mindful living, and specific Ayurvedic techniques, she sought not only to strengthen her vitality but also to experience Ayurveda's promise of a journey toward enlightenment.

Understanding Ojas: The Essence of Digestion

Tara discovered that Ojas is the finest product of digestion, described as a vital essence that sustains strength, mental clarity, and emotional resilience. It flows throughout the body like a nourishing elixir, enhancing immunity and vitality.

However, Tara's weak digestion, fatigue, and inconsistent energy suggested that her Agni (digestive fire) was not functioning optimally, resulting in the accumulation of Ama (toxins) rather than the production of Ojas. Tara committed to an Ayurvedic regimen to strengthen her Agni, enhance Ojas production, and pave the way for experiencing Soma, the spiritual essence linked to higher states of consciousness.

Cultivating Ojas: Nourishment for Body and Mind

Tara realized that to build Ojas, she needed to address three aspects of her lifestyle: diet, stress reduction, and rejuvenation.

Dietary Changes
Tara's diet now included Ojas-building foods like kitchari, ghee, almonds, milk, dates, and fresh, organic fruits and vegetables. These foods not only improved her digestion but also stabilized her mood by supporting serotonin production and enhancing overall emotional well-being.

Strengthening Agni
Tara added warming spices like ginger, cumin, and fennel to her meals, which boosted her digestive fire, transforming food into vital energy and reducing Ama. As her digestion improved, she experienced greater mental clarity, driven by more consistent dopamine regulation.

Daily Abhyanga (Oil Massage)

Tara incorporated daily self-massage with warm herbal oils, which calmed her nervous system, increased circulation, and maintained GABA balance. This practice helped reduce stress and promoted a sense of safety and relaxation.

As Tara's Ojas increased, she noticed enhanced vitality, radiant skin, and improved mood stability. Her physical transformation reflected a deeper harmony between her mind, body, and nervous system.

Soma: Awakening Higher Consciousness

With a stronger foundation of Ojas, Tara felt ready to explore Soma, the refined essence Maharishi described as supporting higher awareness.

> **In Vedic teachings, Soma is produced when the individual reaches higher states of consciousness through the practice of meditation.**

To cultivate Soma, Tara adopted Transcendental Meditation (TM) as a central practice, meditating for 20 minutes twice daily. Her regular practice not only facilitated the production of Soma but also deepened her sense of peace and awareness.

Ojas and Soma: The Real Liquid Intelligence

Tara came to understand that Ojas and Soma were not just theoretical concepts but tangible experiences transforming her health and consciousness.

Physical Vitality

With increased Ojas, Tara's immune system strengthened. She was less prone to illnesses, and her energy remained stable. Balanced neurotransmitters—serotonin, dopamine, and GABA—further supported her physical and mental well-being.

Mental Clarity and Focus

As her nervous system became stress-free, Tara's mental clarity and focus improved. She attributed this to the influence of Ojas, which nourished her ability to transcend ordinary perception and connect with deeper spiritual awareness.

Spiritual Awakening

Tara began to experience unbounded awareness even amidst daily activities, a sign of the growth of higher states of consciousness.

Bridging Ayurveda and Neuroscience

Tara's experiences with Ojas and Soma highlighted the intersection between Ayurveda and modern science.

Serotonin, Dopamine, and GABA

Tara's practices not only increased Ojas and Soma but also balanced key neurotransmitters. Enhanced serotonin improved emotional stability, balanced dopamine fueled motivation and focus, and elevated GABA promoted relaxation and inner peace.

Gut-Brain Connection

Tara understood that strong digestion (Agni) is crucial for both physical and mental clarity. Modern research on the gut-brain axis supported this link, emphasizing that good digestion boosts serotonin production, mood, and immune function—mirroring Ayurveda's teachings on Ojas.

Stress-Free Nervous System

Maharishi's explanation of Soma as the biochemistry of higher consciousness resonated with Tara's experiences. By reducing stress and achieving mental rest, she accessed deeper awareness, bridging physical well-being and spiritual awakening.

Tara's Realization: The Power of Liquid Intelligence

> **Tara realized that Ojas and Soma represent the "real liquid intelligence."**

They embody a holistic approach to well-being, integrating body, mind, and spirit.

By cultivating Ojas and Soma, Tara experienced:

- Stronger Immunity and Vitality

- Enhanced Mental Clarity and Refined Perception

- Emotional Stability and Inner Peace

- Connection to Higher States of Consciousness

Tara's journey demonstrates that Ayurveda's wisdom extends

beyond physical health, offering a pathway to spiritual transformation and the realization of unity in life.

Ojas and Soma: The Pinnacle of Ayurvedic Knowledge

While Ojas and Soma's biochemical nature remains elusive, they symbolize the potential for perfect health and enlightenment, achievable through a holistic integration of body, mind, and spirit. Tara's journey illustrates the profound impact of cultivating these ancient Ayurvedic concepts. They are not just theoretical; they offer a tangible path to total well-being, bridging the timeless wisdom of Ayurveda with the insights of modern neuroscience. Tara's transformation reveals that the pursuit of real liquid intelligence is not only possible but also a pathway to higher states of consciousness.

PART III

STRATEGIES

CHAPTER 16

HABIT CHANGE

The most important strategy to learn is habit change because it teaches you how to adopt all the other protocols in an easy and effective manner. In *16 Super Biohacks for Longevity* and *Neurohacking for Online Learning* we describe a simple process that includes 4 simple concepts to habit change. This process has been enhanced in the *SuperHabits* course (superhabits.com). We will describe the basic concepts here.

- Motivate

- Personalize

- Experiment

- Be Real

Motivate

Motivation is everything. It is hard to learn a new habit if you are not motivated. Motivation can come from fear or inspiration. You could be afraid of getting sick and dying young, and therefore be willing to exercise more. Or, you could be determined to be healthy and fit and thus be inspired to exercise.

> ## Motivation is easier if you have a clear intention.

Some intentions are simple and concrete, others are abstract and all-encompassing. Both are valuable, but habits are generally easier to learn if they are tied to your sense of identity, of who you want to become in your life.

Begin by writing a sentence about something you want to change in your life. Do you want to drink more water? Do you want to become a writer or an artist? It's alright to start with a big idea if you understand that what you are trying to do is create a series of small habits to achieve that bigger goal. Place this statement in the center of a piece of paper or your computer screen as the beginning your Habit Map. For example, "I want to lose 15 pounds over the next three months."

Personalize

Personalize your habits. Each of us needs a different approach to habit change. Ayurveda makes this very clear. If you are a P (Pitta) Energy State person with a strong dopamine drive it's much easier to adopt new habits, but what about others who are not as driven? They need to create strategies that will help them adopt a new habit according to who they are.

Make it personal. You understand that you are part Pitta and part Kapha so you have to find a small habit that will help you achieve this goal. An illustration of the Habit Map and Plan is given below. Around your central goal, in the center of your Habit

Map, like spokes radiating from the hub of a wheel, list some small simple action steps that you believe you can do.

BIOHACK MAP & PLAN

Action Step
Priority
Action Step
Priority
Main Intention or Desire

What is my cue or prompt?
Action Step
How am I measuring success?

Priority
What is my reward?

Taking a 15 minute walk each day could be one idea. Eating fewer calories is another. Maybe eating more slowly and paying more attention on your food would help. Remember, you are part Kapha so your metabolism is little slower than others and you can gain weight easily. You are also part Pitta and tend to eat quickly and may not pay enough attention to the quantity and quality of the food you are eating.

Experiment

Experiment with different approaches. Out of all your ideas on the spokes of your Habit Map, pick one small, specific habit that appeals to you such as, "I am going to eat more slowly and pay more attention to how I am eating the food. I will help myself do this by lowering my fork between each bite of food. I will try this for a month and see how it affects my weight and how I feel." This is your Habit Plan. Instead of rushing through your meal without really savoring it, this new habit will allow you to both taste and appreciate your food more completely.

> **Part of the experiment is finding a *cue* or *prompt* that will help you remember to practice this habit.**

One possible cue might be the act of sitting down and taking your first bite. Another would be to have your partner, a friend, or a family member remind you of this new habit when you sit down. It doesn't have to be a scolding, just a kind reminder in the right direction. You could even have some fun and put a large fork in the center of the table as a cue. Each person needs to find a unique cue that works for them.

Be Real

Be real is a phrase that reminds us that when we transform a strategy into a habit we need constant feedback. How are you going to measure your progress of adopting the new habit of eating more slowly? If you do success for a week what reward will you give yourself. To help you in evaluating your progress we recommend 4 levels of feedback and coaching.

The first is *Self Coaching*. Keep a journal or make notations in your calendar of how well you did for each meal. Whatever is easy for you.

The second is *Partner Coaching*. It also helps to have a buddy who can check in with you and see how you are doing. It may not always be easy to get someone to help you, but it is important. Of course, if you are a P Energy State person you may decide that you have enough willpower to do it yourself, solo. However, having a buddy is an invaluable strategy so at least try it.

Check in with your buddy at the end of the day. If that doesn't work, maybe once a week. The ideal question your buddy can ask you each time is: "Are you doing your best to do your habit?" The answer can be on a scale of 1 to 10. Maybe you had to give yourself a low score for dinner because you had a guest over and got distracted and didn't put your full attention on trying to accomplish this habit. It is alright to have a setback. Talk about all the obstacles and challenges with your buddy. Once things are back to normal, you try again.

Group Coaching is a third level of feedback. If you can create a group to help you with adopting your new habit that is a huge advantage. Many studies have shown group coaching to be highly effective in stopping harmful addictive habits like smoking and alcohol consumption.

Finally, there is *Environmental Coaching*. One obvious example is that if you want to lose weight then you might ask your partner or family if they will support you and remove all the snacks from your home for this time. Changing your environment is an important tool in habit change.

CHAPTER 17

MORNING SUNLIGHT

Sam, a driven 38-year-old tech executive, was no stranger to the relentless grind of modern life. Every day was a blur of packed meetings, relentless deadlines, and constant connectivity that left him feeling drained. His intense work hours and the stress of navigating high-stakes decisions took their toll, with mood swings, restless sleep, and a growing sense of disconnection creeping into his life. Despite his ambition and determination to succeed, Sam felt his energy slipping away, leaving him scattered and unmotivated.

One day, Sam stumbled upon the ancient wisdom of Ayurveda. The idea of aligning his lifestyle with nature's rhythms piqued his curiosity. Among Ayurveda's practices, the concept of dinacharya, or daily routines, caught his attention. Specifically, he was intrigued by the seemingly simple recommendation of basking in morning sunlight. Though skeptical at first, Sam was desperate for a solution—anything to regain his focus, stability, and vitality.

Taking a leap, he embraced this small shift. As he began stepping outside each morning, allowing the gentle rays of dawn to warm his skin, Sam noticed subtle yet profound changes unfolding within him. What he thought was just a minor lifestyle tweak soon blossomed into a powerful transformation, restoring his energy, focus, and overall sense of well-being. Sam's journey with Ayurveda had begun with a simple sunrise, but it promised a brighter future.

Starting the Day: Vata, Dopamine, and Morning Sunlight

Sam's mornings had always been a rush—waking to his phone's alarm, scanning emails, and skipping breakfast to get to work quickly. This chaotic start exacerbated his Vata tendencies, making him feel mentally scattered and anxious.

To address this, Sam set his alarm for 5:30 AM to allow time for a morning routine that included stepping outside at dawn. On his first day, the crisp air and golden rays of the early sun greeted him, bringing an unexpected sense of calm.

Boosting and Regulating Cortisol

Exposure to morning sunlight boosts cortisol production, Cortisol is highly elevated with stress, but at normal levels this hormone is essential for many physiological functions. Sam soon felt more alert, motivated, and mentally clear—qualities that Vata types often struggle to maintain when out of balance.

The sun's warmth also had a grounding effect, calming his nervous system and enhancing his focus. The balanced rise prevented the sudden cortisol spikes that often overwhelmed him during the day.

Calming Vata

Sam found that morning sunlight soothed his anxiety. This practice also regulated his circadian rhythm, improving his sleep quality and leaving him more energized in the mornings.

Balancing Pitta: Cortisol, Serotonin, and Stress Regulation

> **Sam's demanding job often left him feeling burned out, classic signs of Pitta imbalance.**

His drive frequently turned into irritability, and he struggled to unwind after long workdays.

Elevating Serotonin

Over time, early sunlight exposure increased Sam's serotonin production, stabilizing his mood. He became less irritable and experienced a calm sense of well-being. The serotonin boost not only improved his emotional balance but also prevented midday energy slumps.

Cooling Pitta

The gentle rays of the morning sun, combined with a slower start to his day, reduced Sam's internal fire. He felt less reactive and more patient with colleagues and family. The morning sun provided a natural way to regulate his Pitta, allowing him to maintain drive without succumbing to stress.

Invigorating Kapha: Serotonin, Motivation, and Energy Boosts

Although Sam wasn't predominantly Kapha, he still experienced morning lethargy and low motivation, especially during the damp days of late winter and early spring. Ayurveda attributes this sluggishness to an increase in Kapha, which can make it harder to feel energized in the morning.

Elevating Mood and Energy

Morning sunlight served as a natural stimulant. Sam found that a brisk walk in the early sun helped him shake off lethargy and set a positive tone for the day.

Reducing Emotional Stagnation

The natural serotonin increase lifted the feelings of emotional heaviness that Sam often felt during colder months. He became more engaged at work and more connected in personal relationships, with less tendency to withdraw or feel stuck.

Synchronizing Circadian Rhythms: Melanopsin, Melatonin, and Better Sleep

Before starting his morning sunlight routine, Sam struggled with irregular sleep patterns. He often felt wired at night, unable to wind down even when tired. Ayurveda emphasizes Brahma Muhurta (pre-dawn hours) as the ideal time for self-care, aligning the body with natural rhythms.

Melanopsin Activation

The melanopsin receptors in Sam's eyes detected the early light and sent signals to the suprachiasmatic nucleus (SCN), the body's master clock. This reset his internal clock, ensuring melatonin production stopped in the morning and began naturally at night.

Sam's sleep cycle improved, with more restful nights and easier wake-ups.

Improved Sleep Quality

As Sam's circadian rhythms synced with natural light cycles, his overall sleep quality improved. He fell asleep consistently and stayed asleep longer, waking up refreshed. This better sleep contributed to enhanced mood, focus, and energy, creating a positive cycle of well-being.

Morning Sunlight as Real Liquid Intelligence

After a few months of consistent morning sunlight exposure, Sam felt revitalized.

> **The combination of Ayurvedic wisdom and modern neuroscience had helped balance his doshas and optimize neurotransmitter production.**

Mental Clarity

The increased dopamine improved Sam's focus and motivation, qualities he struggled to maintain before. His mornings shifted from chaos and scattered thoughts to calm intention and clear productivity.

Emotional Stability

With higher serotonin levels, Sam experienced greater mood balance and well-being. His reduced irritability allowed him to be more present in both his professional and personal life.

Physical Vitality

Regulated cortisol meant Sam no longer suffered from stress-induced burnout. He had more energy, enthusiasm, and better quality sleep, leading to consistent vitality throughout the day.

Key Takeaways from Sam's Story

Sam's transformation demonstrates how a simple practice like morning sunlight exposure can profoundly impact both body and mind:

- Morning sunlight stimulates dopamine, enhancing focus, motivation, and mental clarity, especially for Vata types.

- Morning sunlight helps regulate cortisol and increase serotonin, reducing stress and mood swings, especially beneficial for Pitta types.

- The early morning sun boosts serotonin, increasing energy and preventing emotional stagnation, particularly important for Kapha types.

- Synchronizing circadian rhythms through morning sunlight improves sleep quality, mood, and overall health.

Morning Sunlight: An Ancient and Modern Biohack

In Ayurveda, morning sunlight is recommended as a way to balance the doshas and connect with nature's rhythms. Modern science confirms that early sunlight positively affects neurotransmitters and hormones, improving mood, energy, and focus. Morning sunlight offers a simple yet powerful way to enhance well-being.

It helps balance Vata, Pitta, and Kapha, ensuring harmony with nature's rhythms.

As an ancient practice endorsed by Ayurveda and validated by modern science, morning sunlight can lead to a healthier, more balanced life. Sam's experience illustrates that aligning with the sun's natural cycles is a profound step toward achieving the real liquid intelligence of mental clarity, emotional balance, and physical vitality.

CHAPTER 18

DIET AND DIGESTION

Kara, a 45-year-old clothing designer known for her vibrant creations, prided herself on her healthy lifestyle. She counted every calorie and carefully tracked nutrients, striving to eat as "clean" as possible. Yet, despite her meticulous approach to food, Kara often found herself feeling anything but balanced. Bloating, sluggishness, and unpredictable mood swings clouded her days, while anxiety and a lack of focus disrupted her creative flow. She began to wonder if there was more to health than just the numbers on a nutrition label.

One day, Kara's curiosity led her to explore Ayurveda. Captivated by the concept of a diet tailored not just to her body, but to her mind and emotions, she sought out an Ayurvedic practitioner. In their first session, she learned she was predominantly Vata-Pitta, with a tendency for Vata imbalances that showed up as anxiety, scattered thoughts, and digestive discomfort. The idea that her unique constitution shaped her response to food felt both fascinating and liberating.

As Kara began her Ayurvedic journey, she was introduced to a whole new way of nourishing herself. It was no longer just about calories or "clean eating" but about cultivating balance and harmony within. She learned the importance of warm, grounding meals and mindful eating practices that soothed her restless Vata nature. With each small adjustment, she noticed her mind growing calmer, her energy more focused, and her creativity flourishing like never before.

This journey wasn't merely about dietary changes—it was an invitation to rediscover herself.

> **Through Ayurveda, Kara found not only relief from her symptoms but a deeper connection to her own well-being, transforming her approach to health from the inside out.**

Understanding Vata Imbalance: From Anxiety to Agni

Kara's practitioner explained that Vata, composed of air and space, governs movement in the body and mind. When Vata becomes imbalanced, it causes anxiety, scattered thoughts, and digestive disturbances like bloating and gas. Kara's habits—skipping meals, eating on the go, and favoring raw salads—aggravated her Vata.

Warm and Nourishing Foods

Kara was advised to switch to warm, cooked meals with grounding ingredients like root vegetables, ghee, and spices like cumin and turmeric. Soups and stews replaced her usual salads, calming her digestive system and reducing bloating.

Dopamine and Vata

The practitioner emphasized that warm, nourishing foods can enhance dopamine production, aiding mental clarity and focus. Tyrosine-rich foods like roasted almonds, avocados, and bananas became staples, helping Kara boost dopamine levels and reduce mental restlessness.

Cooling the Fire: Addressing Pitta Imbalance

While Vata was Kara's primary imbalance, she also had Pitta tendencies, which manifested as irritability, impatience, and occasional heartburn—signs of excess fire in the body.

Cooling and Soothing Foods

Kara added cooling foods like cucumbers, coconut water, and mint to her diet to naturally ease Pitta's heat. She also reduced her intake of caffeine and certain intense flavors that could heighten her irritability. This dietary shift supported more consistent energy levels and helped her avoid the dopamine spikes that often left her feeling drained.

Serotonin and Pitta

Incorporating serotonin-boosting foods like sweet potatoes and walnuts, Kara experienced a steadier mood and noticed her midday irritability easing. These cooling additions kept her Pitta in balance, fostering greater emotional stability and patience throughout her workday.

Balancing Kapha:
Overcoming Lethargy and Stagnation

Although Kapha wasn't her primary dosha, Kara found herself feeling sluggish during the colder months—a sign of Kapha imbalance. Her practitioner explained that while her Vata-Pitta constitution thrived with warmth and grounding foods, the heaviness of winter sometimes called for a subtle shift to keep Kapha in check.

Seasonal Adjustments

To maintain her balance year-round, Kara learned to adjust her diet with the seasons. During the warmer months, she focused on cooling foods to soothe her Pitta. As the weather turned colder, she mindfully introduced moderate amounts of warming spices like ginger, black pepper, and mustard seeds into her meals. These spices helped stimulate her digestion and metabolism, reducing the stagnation she felt in winter, while still respecting her need to avoid overstimulating her Pitta. This careful balancing act allowed her to stay energized and emotionally stable throughout the year.

Applying General Ayurvedic Principles

For each dosha type there are specific recommendations (see Appendix 2). In addition to dosha-specific recommendations, Kara's practitioner emphasized the following general Ayurvedic dietary principles:

Eat Your Largest Meal at Midday

Kara shifted her heaviest meal to lunchtime when her digestive fire (Agni) was strongest. This improved her digestion, energy, and mental clarity throughout the day.

Sit While Eating

Kara made a conscious effort to sit down for meals rather than eat on the go or at her desk. This improved her digestion and left her feeling more satisfied after meals.

Sip Warm Water

Kara sipped warm water throughout the day to support her digestive fire and reduce bloating. The warm water also calmed her Vata, helping her feel grounded.

The Neurotransmitter Connection: Mental Clarity and Emotional Stability

As Kara followed Ayurvedic dietary recommendations over several months, she noticed significant improvements in her mental and emotional state.

Improved Dopamine Levels

Tyrosine-rich foods like avocados, bananas, and almonds maintained her focus and motivation during busy workdays. Kara experienced less scattered energy and more mental clarity.

Balanced Serotonin

Incorporating tryptophan-rich foods like eggs and nuts helped stabilize her mood and reduce anxiety. Her sleep quality also improved, as serotonin is a precursor to melatonin, the sleep hormone.

Enhanced GABA

Foods like spinach, green tea, and brown rice increased GABA levels, reducing anxiety and promoting calm. Kara found it easier to unwind in the evenings and experienced fewer racing thoughts before bed.

Diet as the Foundation of Health

Through Ayurveda, Kara learned that food is not just about physical nourishment but also a pathway to mental and emotional balance.

> **By aligning her diet with her dosha and supporting neurotransmitter production, she discovered a new sense of mental clarity, emotional stability, and physical vitality.**

Mental Clarity

With balanced dopamine levels, Kara felt more focused and productive at work. Her motivation and sense of purpose increased.

Emotional Stability

Serotonin-boosting foods brought calm and contentment, reducing the severe mood swings that had previously troubled her.

Physical Vitality

As her digestion improved, Kara felt more energetic and less weighed down after meals. Her body felt lighter, and her mind clearer, allowing her to approach each day with enthusiasm.

Key Takeaways from Kara's Story

- Warm, grounding foods enhance dopamine levels in Vata types, improving focus and reducing anxiety.

- Cooling, soothing foods balance Pitta, preventing emotional volatility and promoting serotonin production.

- Light, stimulating foods energize Kapha types, boosting dopamine and reducing lethargy.

General Ayurvedic principles—eating the largest meal at midday, sipping warm water, and sitting while eating—support digestion and neurotransmitter balance for all doshas.

Ayurveda's Approach to Diet and Digestion

In Ayurveda, diet is the foundation of health, vitality, and longevity. It emphasizes the importance of strong Agni (digestive fire) for converting food into Ojas (the essence of vitality) and preventing the accumulation of Ama (toxins). Ayurvedic dietary principles aim to balance the doshas and support neurotransmitters like dopamine, serotonin, and GABA, which regulate mood, motivation, and mental clarity.

The Role of Neurotransmitters in Diet

Modern science aligns with Ayurveda's understanding of how food impacts neurotransmitters:

- Dopamine is boosted by tyrosine-rich foods like almonds, avocados, and bananas, which enhance motivation and focus.

- Serotonin is supported by tryptophan-rich foods like turkey, sweet potatoes, and nuts, helping to stabilize mood and improve sleep.

- GABA is enhanced by foods like spinach, green tea, and brown rice, promoting relaxation and reducing anxiety.

By aligning dietary choices with doshic balance and neurotransmitter needs, Ayurveda provides a holistic approach to optimizing mental health.

Diet as the Key to Balance and Longevity

By following a diet that aligns with individual needs, Ayurveda offers a pathway to long-lasting health, mental clarity, and emotional resilience. Kara's story illustrates that the right diet not only supports physical health but also enhances the mind's ability to maintain focus, stability, and vitality. Through a personalized Ayurvedic approach, Kara was able to unlock the full potential of her body and mind, experiencing a new level of well-being.

CHAPTER 19

THE GUT MICROBIOME

Tina, a 45-year-old sales manager with a fast-paced lifestyle, had always been diligent about her health. She stuck to a balanced diet, exercised regularly, and made an effort to manage stress. Yet, despite her commitment, something felt off. Persistent bloating, fatigue, and mood swings shadowed her days, slowly chipping away at her energy and confidence. The symptoms crept into her work life too, making it difficult to stay focused and positive, especially when leading her team.

After months of seeking answers, Tina found herself frustrated, having cycled through several doctors who offered little more than temporary fixes or vague explanations. Desperate for a solution, she finally scheduled an appointment with an Integrative Health specialist known for blending Ayurveda with modern gut health science. From the moment she stepped into the consultation room, Tina sensed this visit might be different.

The doctor introduced her to a concept that would change everything: the gut microbiome. This intricate ecosystem of microorganisms within the digestive system, she learned, played a powerful role not only in digestion but also in immune function and mental health. What fascinated Tina most was the "gut-brain axis"—a communication network between the gut and the brain.

The doctor explained how imbalances in the microbiome could affect neurotransmitter production, fueling anxiety, depression, and even cognitive fog.

For Tina, this was a revelation. Suddenly, her symptoms weren't random; they were connected to an unseen yet influential part of her body. Inspired and eager, she embarked on a tailored wellness plan, incorporating Ayurvedic herbs, gut-healing foods, and lifestyle adjustments designed to nourish her microbiome. Over time, she felt her energy and clarity return, her mood swings settled, and her sense of well-being blossomed.

> **What began as a frustrating search for answers evolved into a journey of discovery—one that redefined health as an intricate balance not just of the body, but of the mind and spirit too.**

Discovering Gut Imbalance: Dysbiosis and Weak Agni

Tina's symptoms suggested an imbalance, or dysbiosis, in her microbiome. A stool test confirmed low levels of beneficial bacteria and an overgrowth of pathogenic strains. The practitioner also noticed signs of weak Agni (digestive fire), a core concept in Ayurveda that, when imbalanced, leads to the accumulation of Ama (toxins) and prevents the creation of Ojas—the vital essence that supports physical and mental resilience.

To restore balance, Tina was given the following holistic plan integrating modern science and Ayurveda.

Probiotics and Prebiotics

Tina began taking a daily probiotic supplement to replenish beneficial bacteria, while increasing prebiotic foods like garlic, onions, and bananas to feed the good bacteria.

Ayurvedic Dietary Adjustments

Her diet was tailored to include more Ojas-building foods—nourishing and easy-to-digest options like kitchari, ghee, and cooked vegetables. These foods also helped reduce the production of Ama.

Agni Stimulation

To strengthen her Agni, Tina drank warm water with fresh ginger each morning. This simple practice ignited her digestive fire and improved nutrient absorption.

Triphala Supplementation

She took Triphala, an Ayurvedic herbal blend known for its gentle detoxifying effects, to cleanse and rejuvenate the gut lining.

Cultivating Vitality and Emotional Balance

As Tina's digestion improved, she began to experience the following benefits:

Reduced Bloating and Fatigue

Within a few weeks, Tina noticed a significant reduction in bloating and an increase in energy levels. This was a clear sign that her Agni was stronger and that her gut flora was more balanced.

Mood Stabilization

The boost in beneficial bacteria led to increased serotonin and dopamine production, which improved Tina's mood and motivation. She felt more emotionally resilient and less prone to the anxiety and mood swings that had plagued her.

Improved Sleep

As her gut health improved, Tina also experienced better sleep quality, likely due to balanced serotonin levels—essential for melatonin production and a healthy sleep-wake cycle.

Bridging Ayurveda and Modern Gut Health

Tina's journey highlighted the profound connection between gut health and mental well-being.

Gut Microbiome and Neurotransmitters

The beneficial bacteria in Tina's gut influenced the production of key neurotransmitters like serotonin and dopamine, regulating mood and emotional stability. Her experience aligned with modern research on the gut-brain axis, which emphasizes the microbiome's role in mental health.

Strong Agni for Ojas Production

In Ayurveda, strong digestion is crucial for creating Ojas, the essence of vitality and resilience. Modern science supports this concept by showing that a well-functioning gut promotes nutrient absorption and overall health.

Ayurveda and the Microbiome

Ayurveda's ancient principles align closely with modern understandings of the gut microbiome. In Ayurveda, maintaining a balanced digestive system is seen as the key to preventing disease and promoting longevity. Ayurveda locates the seat of Vata in the colon, which contains the largest portion of the gut microbiome. Vata is responsible for the functioning of the nervous system and the gut microbiome is part of the gut-brain axis.

Ayurveda recommends consuming natural probiotics, such as lassi (a drink made from yogurt, water, and spices), to support digestion. Periodic detoxification, such as panchakarma, helps remove Ama and reset the digestive system, allowing the gut to heal and the microbiome to rebalance. By following Ayurvedic dietary guidelines tailored to individual doshas, we can support a healthy microbiome and prevent the imbalances that lead to disease.

> **Ayurveda's wisdom about the importance of digestion and its modern counterpart—microbiome research—both point to the same conclusion: a healthy gut is the foundation of a healthy body and mind.**

By nurturing our microbiome through diet, probiotics, prebiotics, and periodic detoxification, we can maintain balance, prevent disease, and support both physical and mental well-being throughout our lives.

Gut Health as the Gateway to Vitality

By focusing on her gut health, Tina was able to enhance both her physical vitality and mental clarity. She came to understand that gut health is not just about digestion but also about the production of vital substances like Ojas and Soma, which integrate the body, mind, and spirit.

Enhanced Vitality

Tina felt stronger and more resilient, with fewer physical ailments and a greater sense of overall well-being.

Mental Clarity and Focus

Balanced dopamine levels improved her concentration and productivity, allowing her to excel at work.

Emotional Stability

Increased serotonin and GABA production brought a sense of calm and emotional balance, reducing mood swings and anxiety.

Spiritual Growth

With regular meditation and reduced stress, Tina experienced deeper spiritual awareness with a more balanced level of neurotransmitters.

Key Takeaways from Tina's Story

Restoring gut health through probiotics, prebiotics, and Ayurvedic dietary practices can improve neurotransmitter production and overall vitality. Strong Agni is essential for the production of Ojas, which sustains physical health, mental clarity, and emotional stability.

Meditation and stress reduction enable the production of Soma, the refined biochemistry of higher consciousness. The integration of Ayurveda and modern science provides a comprehensive approach to health, addressing both physical and mental well-being.

CHAPTER 20

SUPPLEMENTS

Mark, a 38-year-old architect with a reputation for his quick thinking and razor-sharp instincts, was used to tackling complex problems with ease. He loved the thrill of designing sleek skyscrapers and tackling last-minute client requests. But over time, the relentless pace began to take its toll.

As project deadlines stacked up, Mark noticed subtle changes creeping in. His once laser-like focus was starting to blur. His mornings stretched into foggy afternoons, with coffee barely propping him up. By evening, irritability took hold, making him snap at friends and family. And when he tried to sleep, he'd lie there wide awake, mind racing with unfinished tasks, feeling "wired" but too drained to accomplish anything. It was a vicious cycle that left him exhausted, yet oddly restless.

Desperate for a solution, Mark tried every trick he could think of—cutting back on caffeine, squeezing in breaks, even starting a meditation practice. Though these changes offered a bit of relief, his focus and energy remained elusive. Frustration grew as he realized that his go-to methods just weren't enough.

Finally, he decided to seek outside help. A friend suggested he see a holistic health practitioner. With some hesitation, Mark made the appointment, hoping that maybe—just maybe—a new approach could help him find his balance and regain the clarity he once took for granted.

Understanding Mark's Imbalances: Dopamine and GABA

The practitioner noted that Mark's symptoms were likely linked to imbalances in dopamine and GABA, two critical neurotransmitters.

> **Dopamine, responsible for motivation, focus, and mood regulation, was depleted by Mark's demanding job and high stress.**

Low dopamine levels led to mental fog, reduced motivation, and feelings of burnout. On the other hand, GABA, which promotes relaxation and calmness, was also low, leaving Mark feeling anxious and unable to unwind or sleep properly.

Integrating Modern Supplements with Ayurvedic Wisdom

To address these issues, the practitioner suggested a supplement regimen integrating modern supplements with Ayurvedic herbs to restore neurotransmitter balance and promote overall well-being. Here are some of the most popular and well-known supplements:

L-Tyrosine
This amino acid is a precursor to dopamine, supporting its production and boosting focus and motivation. Within a week of starting L-Tyrosine, Mark noticed a sharper focus and increased motivation at work.

Rhodiola Rosea

An adaptogenic herb known to reduce fatigue and support both dopamine and serotonin levels. Rhodiola helped Mark manage stress more effectively, preventing the mental burnout that had been draining his energy.

GABA Supplement

Taken in the evening, the GABA supplement promoted relaxation, reduced anxiety, and improved sleep quality. Mark began sleeping more soundly, with fewer episodes of restlessness and anxiety at night.

Omega-3 Fatty Acids

The fish oil supplements, rich in Omega-3s, supported brain function, dopamine production, and mood stability. After a few weeks, Mark experienced more consistent energy and improved mental clarity.

Adding Ayurvedic Practices for Comprehensive Healing

As Mark's energy and mental clarity improved, he became interested in incorporating more Ayurvedic practices into his routine.

Triphala

Mark added this Ayurvedic blend to support his gut health, indirectly boosting serotonin production for better mood stability.

Ashwagandha

This Ayurvedic adaptogen reduced stress and increased serotonin production, calming Mark's nervous system. It also helped regulate cortisol, preventing the highs and lows of stress. Mark felt less irritable and noticed a more stable mood throughout the day.

Brahmi (Bacopa Monnieri)
He also started taking Brahmi to improve memory and concentration. By combining modern supplements with Ayurvedic herbs, Mark was able to address his neurotransmitter imbalances holistically.

The Role of Supplements in Mental and Physical Health

Supplements have gained popularity as tools for enhancing mental clarity, energy, and overall vitality. They work by providing the necessary precursors, cofactors, or support for neurotransmitter production and function. Let's explore how various supplements target different neurotransmitters.

Dopamine-Enhancing Supplements

L-Tyrosine: As a precursor to dopamine, it supports focus, energy, and mood. Studies suggest that L-Tyrosine can improve cognitive performance, especially during stress.

Rhodiola Rosea: This adaptogen reduces fatigue, enhances mental performance, and balances dopamine and serotonin levels.

Mucuna Pruriens: Also known as the velvet bean, it contains L-DOPA, a direct precursor to dopamine. Research shows it is effective in increasing dopamine, improving mood, and supporting motor function.

Serotonin-Enhancing Supplements

Tryptophan: A precursor to serotonin and can reduce symptoms of depression and anxiety.

St. John's Wort: Used for centuries to treat mild to moderate depression, it boosts serotonin but should be used cautiously due to potential interactions with medications.

SAM-e: A naturally occurring compound that supports neurotransmitter production, SAM-e has shown promise in improving mood by enhancing both serotonin and dopamine.

GABA-Enhancing Supplements

GABA Supplement: Direct supplementation with GABA can promote relaxation, reduce anxiety, and improve sleep.

L-Theanine: Found in green tea, L-Theanine increases GABA levels, promoting relaxation without drowsiness and improving mental focus.

Ayurvedic Supplements for Holistic Health

Ayurveda offers herbal remedies that complement modern supplements and target both mental clarity and physical vitality:

Triphala: This blend supports gut health, indirectly boosting serotonin production through the gut-brain axis.

Ashwagandha: As an adaptogen, it reduces stress by increasing serotonin levels and lowering cortisol, promoting a sense of calm.

Brahmi (Bacopa Monnieri): Brahmi enhances memory, learning, and concentration by increasing acetylcholine production, essential for cognitive health.

Turmeric (Curcumin): With anti-inflammatory properties, turmeric boosts brain-derived neurotrophic factor (BDNF), improving neuroplasticity and supporting serotonin and dopamine levels.

General Supplements

There are hundreds of supplements sold to improve physical and mental energy, reduce inflammation, and promote overall vitality. One simple recommendation is to take a daily vitamin and mineral supplement. More specific recommendations might include:

Magnesium: Essential for muscle relaxation, energy production, and GABA balance, magnesium helps reduce anxiety and promote restful sleep.

Omega-3 Fatty Acids: These fatty acids support brain health, cardiovascular health, and neurotransmitter production, improving mood and reducing anxiety.

Coenzyme Q10 (CoQ10): A powerful antioxidant that supports cellular energy production and protects against oxidative damage, CoQ10 is particularly beneficial for aging and heart health.

Key Takeaways

Supplements can restore neurotransmitter balance, improving focus, mood, and relaxation. Integrating modern supplements with Ayurvedic herbs offers a comprehensive approach to mental and physical well-being. Personalized supplement regimens can address specific neurotransmitter imbalances, supporting overall vitality.

By supporting neurotransmitter balance, reducing stress, and promoting overall vitality, supplements—both modern and Ayurvedic—offer powerful tools for enhancing well-being. As seen in Mark's journey, an integrated supplement regimen can restore focus, energy, and mood while also providing a foundation for long-term health and balance.

CHAPTER 21

DETOX

Amelia, a vibrant 45-year-old woman, had always been the heart of her home, infusing every room with warmth and positivity. Her days were a flurry of activity—cooking family meals, managing household chores, planning outings—all with her usual energy and cheer. But over the past year, something had shifted. Amelia began to feel unusually sluggish and mentally foggy, her mind often clouded in a haze that even a good night's sleep couldn't clear.

Despite following a diet she'd always believed to be healthy, her body felt out of sync. Mornings that once greeted her with a sense of renewal now seemed heavy and uninviting. Bloating became a daily frustration, and her moods seemed to turn on a dime, flipping from irritability to anxiety with little warning. Friends and family began noticing the changes, and she could feel herself withdrawing, desperate for answers but uncertain where to turn.

Feeling lost, Amelia decided to try a different approach. She sought out an Ayurvedic practitioner, intrigued by the promise of a more holistic perspective. During their first meeting, the practitioner listened intently, connecting her symptoms to an imbalance of Kapha and a buildup of Ama—toxins her body couldn't rid itself of, disrupting her digestion and clouding her mind.

The practitioner proposed a personalized detox regimen, one designed to clear her system of Ama and restore harmony to her doshas. With each step of this new journey, Amelia could feel the fog lifting, a clarity returning that she had almost forgotten. Slowly, the warmth and energy she'd always been known for began to re-emerge, filling her with a renewed sense of vitality and emotional balance.

Amelia's Detox Program: A Multi-Level Approach

> **Amelia's detox plan was structured around daily, weekly, and seasonal practices, creating a holistic path toward cleansing and rejuvenation.**

Daily Detox Routine: Laying the Foundation

Morning Hydration
Each morning, Amelia drank a glass of water upon waking, a simple practice that improved digestion and regularity. This helped her eliminate toxins more effectively.

Meditation and Light Exercise
Before breakfast, Amelia practiced Transcendental Meditation (TM) for 20 minutes, calming her mind and enhancing dopamine production. Following TM, she performed light yoga, which boosted circulation, supported digestion, and elevated her

energy levels.

Meals and Digestive Aids

Amelia followed an elimination diet, which revealed that gluten was contributing to her digestive discomfort. She made lunch her largest meal, ate slowly, and sipped warm water throughout the day to support Agni (digestive fire). To stimulate digestion, Amelia drank a pre-meal tonic of ginger juice, lemon, and a pinch of salt before lunch and dinner.

Digestive Tea

Throughout the day, she sipped a tea made from cumin, fennel, and coriander seeds, which aided in flushing toxins and balancing digestion.

Triphala at Bedtime

Before bed, Amelia took Triphala with warm water, which supported regular elimination, stabilized serotonin levels, and improved her sleep quality.

Weekly Detox: Liquid Day for Rest and Reset

Each Saturday, Amelia dedicated a day to liquid detox. She consumed light broths and herbal teas, allowing her digestive system to rest. This practice reduced Ama and Kapha congestion, leading to a lighter body and clearer mind.

Spring Detox: Kitchari Cleanse for Deep Cleansing

As spring approached, Amelia embarked on a more intensive Kitchari cleanse. For five days, Amelia ate kitchari—a simple dish made from mung beans, rice, and spices—at all meals to reset her digestion and eliminate toxins. Her Kapha-reducing diet emphasized light, bitter, and astringent foods like leafy greens, while avoiding heavy, oily foods.

After the cleanse, Amelia felt light, energized, and more mentally clear. Her mood improved, and she experienced a renewed sense of optimism and stability.

Panchakarma: The Ultimate Ayurvedic Detox

At the end of summer, Amelia decided to undergo Panchakarma, Ayurveda's most comprehensive detoxification therapy, including:

Virechana (Purgation)
This herbal purgation helped cleanse Amelia's liver and gut, releasing deep-seated Ama.

Abhyanga (Oil Massage) and Swedana (Steam Therapy)
Oil massages and steam therapy helped loosen toxins, improved circulation, and promoted relaxation.

Basti (Medicated Enemas)
Basti supported her gut health, which was essential for balancing serotonin and dopamine production.

Nasya (Nasal Administration of Oils)
Nasya cleared Amelia's sinuses and soothed her nervous system, enhancing her mental clarity.

Results of Detox: Amelia's Transformation

After completing her detox program, Amelia noticed some remarkable changes:

Increased Energy
Her energy levels soared, replacing the sluggishness she had previously felt.

Mental Clarity
The mental fog lifted, leading to sharper focus and clearer thinking.

Stable Mood
Her mood swings diminished, resulting in consistent emotional well-being.

Regular Digestion
Amelia's digestion became more regular, leaving her feeling lighter and more comfortable.

The Power of Ayurvedic Detox

Ayurveda's detox practices emphasize removing toxins, restoring doshic balance, and enhancing the production of key neurotransmitters for mental clarity and emotional resilience. Unlike extreme detox diets, Ayurveda offers a sustainable and natural approach that aligns with the body's rhythms, promoting overall well-being.

Daily, weekly, and seasonal detox practices offer a sustainable path to maintaining vitality and mental clarity. Panchakarma provides a deep reset, balancing the doshas and enhancing overall health. Amelia's story illustrates the profound impact of detox on achieving greater energy, sharper focus, and emotional resilience, demonstrating how cleansing the body can also lead to a clearer, more vibrant mind.

CHAPTER 22

SLEEP

Liam, a dynamic 32-year-old product manager, was known for his tireless drive and unwavering dedication to his work. He thrived on the excitement of product launches and project deadlines, his energy and focus an inspiration to his team. But as the months wore on, Liam's seemingly endless stamina began to falter. Nights that once offered him restful sleep transformed into a frustrating battle; he would lie in bed exhausted yet unable to drift off. And even if he did manage to sleep, he would often wake around 2 or 3 a.m., feeling restless and uncomfortably warm, unable to quiet his mind and return to slumber.

As these sleepless nights stacked up, they began to take a toll. His mood grew irritable, his focus wavered, and the sharpness that had always defined his work started to blur. Liam tried all the typical sleep aids—cutting down on late caffeine, winding down with soothing music, even trying melatonin—but nothing seemed to break the cycle. His body was tired, but his mind refused to follow suit.

Fed up, Liam decided to seek an alternative solution and scheduled a visit with an Ayurvedic practitioner. During their consultation, the practitioner carefully listened to Liam's symptoms, linking them to imbalances in his Pitta and Vata doshas.

The excess Pitta energy, he explained, was generating an inner restlessness, while an unsteady Vata was fueling Liam's erratic sleep patterns, leaving him unable to stay asleep.

Eager to reclaim his vitality, Liam took his practitioner's advice and adopted a tailored Ayurvedic sleep routine. This included grounding rituals to calm his Vata and cooling practices to pacify his Pitta before bed. With each night, the balance he'd lost began to return.

Gradually, Liam found himself falling asleep with ease, staying asleep through the night, and waking up feeling truly refreshed—ready to tackle the day once again with his signature energy and focus.

Understanding Liam's Sleep Struggles

Liam's primary sleep issues included:

Difficulty falling asleep
Work stress kept his dopamine levels high, making his mind active well into the night.

Frequent waking between 2-3 am
This is a classic sign of Pitta imbalance, often caused by overheating or overstimulation.

Fatigue and irritability
Erratic sleep disrupted serotonin and melatonin regulation, leading to irritability and lack of focus.

Liam's New Ayurvedic Sleep Routine

To restore balance, the Ayurvedic practitioner introduced Liam to the following holistic sleep routine:

Evening Wind-Down
Right before dinner, Liam practiced Transcendental Meditation (TM) for 20 minutes, calming his mind and balancing dopamine and serotonin.

He opted for a light, cooling dinner featuring cucumber salad, leafy greens, and basmati rice to pacify Pitta and prevent night-time overheating.

Warm Bath with Essential Oils
Around 8:30 p.m., Liam took a warm bath infused with lavender oil. The warmth relaxed his muscles, while the lavender scent promoted GABA release, encouraging relaxation.

Golden Milk for Vata
About 30 minutes before bed, Liam sipped golden milk (warm milk with turmeric and honey). This calming drink helped ground his Vata energy, preparing him for sleep.

Tech-Free Time
Liam turned off screens an hour before bed, as blue light inhibited melatonin production. This helped him wind down more naturally.

Regular Bedtime
Liam committed to a consistent sleep schedule, going to bed by 10:00 p.m. and waking at 6:00 a.m., aligning with natural

circadian rhythms. This helped stabilize serotonin and dopamine levels, making his sleep more restorative.

Morning Sunlight Exposure
Liam started spending 15 minutes in natural sunlight shortly after waking, boosting dopamine and cortisol production, which improved his energy and mental clarity.

Results of Liam's Sleep Routine

Within weeks, Liam experienced these significant improvements:

Easier sleep onset
The calming pre-bed routine quieted his mind, making it easier to fall asleep.

Fewer nighttime awakenings
Cooling his evening routine and meals reduced his 2-3 a.m. wake-ups.

Improved mood and focus
With consistent, restorative sleep, Liam felt more stable emotionally and more focused at work.

The Science of Sleep: Neurotransmitters at Play

Sleep affects mental, physical, and emotional health, mainly through neurotransmitter regulation. The key neurotransmitters involved in sleep include:

Melatonin

Produced by the pineal gland, melatonin regulates the sleep-wake cycle. It rises with darkness, preparing the body for rest.

Dopamine

While primarily known for motivation and wakefulness, dopamine also affects sleep quality. Elevated dopamine levels in the evening can delay sleep onset, while balanced levels support deeper rest.

Serotonin

This precursor to melatonin plays a vital role in mood stability and sleep. Low serotonin levels can disrupt sleep patterns and contribute to insomnia.

GABA

As the brain's primary inhibitory neurotransmitter, GABA calms neural activity, promoting sleep and reducing anxiety.

The Glymphatic System: Detox During Sleep

During sleep, the brain's glymphatic system becomes active, clearing away toxins like beta-amyloid plaques, which are associated with conditions like Alzheimer's disease. This detoxification process peaks during deep sleep, emphasizing the importance of achieving restorative rest. Disrupted sleep can impair this system, increasing the risk of cognitive decline.

Sleep Supplements: Supporting Better Rest

Melatonin supplements can help some people regulate sleep-wake cycles, especially for those with difficulty falling asleep, but recent research suggests a lower dose may be more effective. Factors like artificial light, stress, and aging can reduce natural melatonin production.

Magnesium, tryptophan, valerian, L-Theanine, and ginkgo biloba have varying effects on promoting relaxation and improving sleep quality.

Ayurvedic Sleep Recommendations: Tailoring to Your Dosha

Ayurveda emphasizes that sleep quality is deeply connected to one's dosha.

Vata

▍ Sleep Challenges: Vata types often have restless minds, leading to insomnia or fragmented sleep.

▍ Sleep Tips: Calming routines, warm baths, golden milk, and soothing sounds can help Vata individuals fall asleep and stay asleep.

Pitta

▍ Sleep Challenges: Pitta types often wake up in the middle of the night, especially around 2-3 a.m., due to overheating or overthinking.

▍ Sleep Tips: Cooling routines, avoiding spicy foods, and

engaging in calming activities before bed help pacify Pitta energy and promote uninterrupted sleep.

Kapha

Sleep Challenges: Kapha types may oversleep and struggle with morning grogginess.

Sleep Tips: Early rising, morning exercise, and lighter evening meals can prevent heaviness and promote energy.

General Recommendations for Optimal Sleep

Regardless of dosha, Ayurveda recommends:

Consistent Sleep Routine

Going to bed by 10:00 p.m. and waking up by 6:00 a.m. aligns with natural circadian rhythms, promoting balanced neurotransmitter production.

Calming Evening Rituals

Light meals, warm baths, and calming activities like reading or stretching encourage serotonin to convert to melatonin, signaling the body to rest.

Reducing blue light exposure by limiting screen time in the evening helps maintain healthy melatonin levels, promoting better sleep quality.

The Power of Ayurvedic Sleep Practices

Prioritizing sleep is one of the most effective ways to support mental and physical health. Whether it's through lifestyle adjustments, supplements, or Ayurvedic practices, focusing on sleep can significantly enhance well-being. Liam's story demonstrates how addressing sleep through an Ayurvedic lens can improve energy, focus, and mood, allowing for more restful and rejuvenating sleep.

Integrating Ayurvedic sleep practices, along with an understanding of how neurotransmitters influence rest, can provide a holistic approach to achieving restorative sleep, mental clarity, and emotional balance.

CHAPTER 23

EXERCISE

Nia, a 45-year-old university administrator, was known for her tireless dedication to her work. She managed a heavy workload with poise, juggling endless meetings, emails, and deadlines. But behind her professional demeanor, Nia was struggling. Her fast-paced life was ironically marked by long hours at her desk, and over the years, a sedentary lifestyle took its toll. She began to notice gradual but stubborn weight gain, a lack of energy, and a creeping sense of anxiety that lingered throughout her day. Though she knew that exercise could help, finding the motivation to start felt like an impossible challenge.

Determined to break free from this cycle, Nia reached out to an Ayurvedic practitioner, hoping to find a new approach. In her consultation, she was surprised to learn that her primary dosha was Kapha. Known for its steady, grounding energy, Kapha also has a tendency to slide into sluggishness, weight gain, and low motivation when out of balance. The practitioner explained that this imbalance was likely the root cause of her physical and mental heaviness, a weight that wasn't just physical but also affected her mood and sense of vitality.

With this understanding, Nia's practitioner suggested a personalized plan to get her moving—a regimen that would honor her Kapha nature while encouraging lightness and energy. She was encouraged to start small but stay consistent, choosing invigorating activities that would break through the inertia, like brisk walks, gentle morning yoga, and a diet to reignite her natural vitality.

> **Inspired by this tailored approach, Nia began to incorporate these changes, and soon, her energy levels started to shift.**

Her days felt a little lighter, her mood brighter, and even the smallest workouts brought a spark of motivation she hadn't felt in years. For the first time, she felt empowered to move her body with purpose, setting in motion a journey to reclaim her health and vibrancy.

Understanding Nia's Exercise Challenges

Nia's struggles with exercise included:

Low energy and motivation
Despite feeling tired during the day, she struggled to initiate any form of exercise.

Weight gain and sluggishness
Her Kapha constitution, coupled with a sedentary lifestyle, led to a feeling of heaviness and inertia.

Increased anxiety
Lack of movement prevented her body from releasing tension and boosting mood-enhancing neurotransmitters.

Nia's New Ayurvedic Exercise Routine

The practitioner designed an exercise regimen tailored to Nia's Kapha constitution, focusing on invigorating and energizing activities that would enhance her metabolism and increase motivation.

Morning Walks in Sunlight
Nia started her day with a 20-minute brisk walk in morning sunlight. This routine stimulated dopamine and endorphin release, helping to energize her Kapha dosha. The fresh air and sunlight also lifted her mood and provided a burst of energy, setting a positive tone for the day.

Incorporating Variety
To prevent boredom, Nia's routine included a mix of exercises: jogging, dancing, and tennis. Each session lasted 30-45 minutes, providing cardiovascular benefits and sustaining consistent dopamine release.

Strength Training
Twice a week, Nia added strength training to build muscle and boost her metabolism. This dynamic exercise helped prevent Kapha stagnation and promoted mental alertness.

Group Classes for Social Interaction

Nia joined a weekly dance class, finding joy in the movement and the social engagement. The combination of physical activity and social interaction released endorphins and lifted her spirits.

Cooling Exercises to Balance Pitta

Given her secondary Pitta traits, such as competitiveness and a tendency to overheat, the practitioner recommended swimming twice a week. This cooling exercise helped maintain balance and prevent burnout.

Yoga for Recovery

On her rest days, Nia practiced gentle yoga to maintain flexibility, reduce anxiety, and balance her doshas. This recovery routine aligned with Ayurveda's approach to nurturing the body after intense physical exertion.

Results of Nia's Exercise Routine

Within a few months, Nia experienced dramatic changes:

Increased energy and motivation

Morning walks and varied exercises helped break Kapha inertia. She felt lighter and more motivated throughout the day.

Weight loss and reduced sluggishness

Regular strength training and vigorous activities helped reduce her weight and feelings of heaviness.

Improved mood and reduced anxiety

The release of dopamine and endorphins from regular exercise led to fewer anxiety episodes and an overall positive outlook.

The Importance of Exercise

Exercise is essential for overall health, reducing the risk of chronic conditions such as cardiovascular disease, type 2 diabetes, obesity, and depression. Studies show that regular physical activity:

▌ Improves muscle strength, endurance, flexibility, and balance.

▌ Prevents the buildup of visceral fat, which contributes to metabolic disorders.

▌ Enhances brain function by promoting neurogenesis, improving mood, and boosting memory.

Exercise, Neurotransmitters, and Mental Health

> **Exercise has profound effects on the brain, improving mood, focus, and emotional resilience.**

It stimulates the production of key neurotransmitters:

Dopamine

Regular physical activity helps regulate the dopamine control circuit, boosting motivation and focus. This is particularly important for managing the dopamine imbalances of Kapha types.

Serotonin

Exercise enhances serotonin production, contributing to mood stability, reducing anxiety, and improving sleep quality.

GABA

The primary inhibitory neurotransmitter, GABA promotes relaxation. Exercise increases GABA levels, calming the nervous system.

Endorphins

Known as "feel-good" chemicals, endorphins reduce pain and increase feelings of pleasure.

Ayurvedic Perspectives on Exercise

In Ayurveda, exercise is an essential component of maintaining health, but the type, intensity, and duration depend on one's dosha.

Vata

Characteristics: Vata types are quick, energetic, but prone to inconsistency and fatigue.

Recommended Exercises: Walking, cycling, dancing, and gentle yoga. Activities should be moderate to avoid exhaustion, as Vata types can tire easily.

Focus: Vata individuals should engage in warm, grounding, and rhythmic exercises to promote stability and prevent anxiety.

Pitta

Characteristics: Pitta types are strong, competitive, and goal-oriented but may overheat or push themselves too hard.

Recommended Exercises: Swimming, hiking, skiing, and team sports. Cooling activities are especially beneficial.

Focus: Pitta types should prioritize relaxing, cooling exercises to prevent overheating and burnout.

Kapha

Characteristics: Kapha types are naturally strong, with good endurance, but may be prone to lethargy.

Recommended Exercises: Running, jogging, strength training, and vigorous sports like tennis. These exercises promote energy and reduce Kapha's heaviness.

Focus: Kapha individuals should choose invigorating, energizing activities that prevent stagnation and boost metabolism.

General Recommendations for All Doshas

Morning Movement

Engaging in physical activity early in the day helps stabilize neurotransmitter levels and aligns with natural circadian rhythms.

Variety and Consistency

Incorporating a range of activities—cardio, strength training, and flexibility exercises—helps maintain physical and mental balance.

Balancing Intensity: Listen to your body
Push yourself enough to build strength and endurance, but avoid overexertion, which can cause imbalances.

Exercise as a Path to Balance and Longevity

For Nia, integrating regular exercise into her routine led to better energy, mood, and physical health. By addressing her Kapha imbalance with invigorating physical activities, she experienced a profound shift in both body and mind.

> **Exercise is not only a prescription for physical health but also a powerful tool for mental well-being.**

Whether you begin with a simple walk or engage in more intense forms of exercise, moving your body is one of the most effective ways to enhance your overall well-being. Through the lens of Ayurveda, exercise becomes not just a daily task but a vital practice for maintaining balance and achieving optimal health.

CHAPTER 24

HYDRATION AND
COLD THERAPY

D r. Lauren Mitchell, a seasoned marine biologist, was no stranger to adventure. Her research took her to the ocean's hidden depths, where she would dive into unknown waters, uncovering the mysteries of marine ecosystems. Lauren's days were filled with physically demanding dives, data collection, and navigating remote areas where access to fresh water was often scarce. She thrived in these challenging conditions, her mental acuity sharp and her body well-conditioned for her demanding fieldwork.

But lately, Lauren had begun to notice subtle but concerning changes. After long dives, her energy waned, her head ached, and her usually sharp focus blurred. As a scientist, she knew the importance of hydration, especially under the sun and after hours in the ocean. Yet, engrossed in her work, she often neglected her own needs, pushing hydration aside to save time.

When her symptoms persisted, Lauren suspected she was experiencing chronic dehydration—a silent yet powerful enemy that could undermine her health and research. Determined to make a change, she delved into a new approach. Drawing from both Ayurvedic wisdom and modern biohacks, she crafted a hydration strategy tailored to her unique lifestyle. She added natural electrolytes, sipped warm water throughout the day to support digestion, and incorporated cold-water immersion to enhance circulation and vitality.

With each dive, Lauren felt a renewed sense of resilience. Her energy sustained her throughout the long hours, her mind was clear, and her body felt balanced even after the most challenging dives. Embracing this new approach to self-care, Lauren realized that nourishing her own well-being was just as important as protecting the ocean she loved.

Lauren's New Hydration Routine

Lauren's efforts to improve her energy levels and mental clarity involved several key adjustments. Lauren set reminders on her diving watch to drink water regularly throughout the day. She carried a special thermos to maintain the water's cool temperature, making it more refreshing after dives.

She started each morning with a glass of room temperature water and a squeeze of lime to kickstart her hydration.

Cold-Water Immersion for Recovery

Lauren's mentor, an experienced diver, suggested cold-water immersion as a recovery tool. Initially hesitant, Lauren began with brief cold showers and gradually added cold plunges in the ocean after dives.

She experienced improved alertness, mood, and focus after these cold sessions, feeling mentally recharged and physically invigorated.

Ayurvedic Insights for Pitta Balance

Consulting with an Ayurvedic practitioner, Lauren learned that her Pitta nature—characterized by high energy and intensity—required cool or room-temperature water, particularly in warm climates.

She began drinking mint-infused water throughout the day to keep her Pitta energy balanced and prevent overheating.

The Results: Lauren's Transformation

After implementing consistent hydration and cold therapy, Lauren noticed significant improvements such as:

Enhanced Cognitive Performance
Regular hydration and cold plunges boosted her mental clarity during dives, allowing her to make quick decisions with ease.

Reduced Fatigue
Proper hydration helped her combat dehydration-induced fatigue, while cold-water immersion increased her dopamine and serotonin levels, uplifting her mood.

Improved Physical Endurance
The combination of hydration and cold exposure increased her stamina and ability to recover from demanding dives, both physically and mentally.

Hydration: The Foundation of Brain and Body Health

Water makes up about 60% of the human body and is critical for almost every physiological function. Beyond hydration, water plays a significant role in regulating neurotransmitters that influence mood, focus, and overall well-being. Proper hydration is essential for:

Cognitive Function
Water keeps brain cells hydrated, which is crucial for maintaining mental clarity, concentration, and focus. Dehydration can reduce cognitive performance, leading to irritability, fatigue, and impaired decision-making.

Muscle Strength and Recovery
Muscles rely on water for proper contraction, and dehydration can result in weakness, cramping, and slower recovery.

Detoxification
Organs like the liver and kidneys depend on water to flush out toxins, maintaining balance and preventing the buildup of harmful substances.

Temperature Regulation
Water helps regulate body temperature through sweating and respiration, which is especially important during physical exertion or in warm environments.

Hydration and Neurotransmitters

Proper hydration is not only vital for physical health but also for optimizing neurotransmitter balance.

Dopamine
Adequate hydration helps maintain healthy dopamine levels, improving motivation and focus.

Serotonin
Water supports serotonin production, which is crucial for mood stability and emotional balance.

GABA
Hydration aids in GABA production, promoting relaxation and stress relief.

Dosha-Specific Hydration: Ayurveda's Perspective

> **Ayurveda offers a personalized approach to hydration based on the doshas—Vata, Pitta, and Kapha. Each dosha has unique hydration needs.**

Vata
Vata types are prone to dryness and dehydration. They benefit from sipping warm water throughout the day to prevent imbalance. Recommendation: 6-8 cups of warm water daily, evenly distributed to support digestion.

Pitta

Pitta types tend to overheat, making cool or room temperature water essential for balance. Recommendation: 8-10 cups of cool or room temperature water daily, especially in warm weather or after physical activity.

Kapha

Kapha types can retain water easily, so they benefit from moderate hydration with warm or room temperature water to prevent stagnation. Recommendation: 8-10 cups of water daily, avoiding cold water that could increase heaviness.

Cold-Water Immersion: Enhancing Brain Chemistry

Cold-water immersion, often referred to as cold therapy, has emerged as a powerful tool for boosting neurotransmitter levels and promoting longevity.

> **Be sure to check with your health provider to make sure they feel this type of therapy will be good for your particular health conditions.**

By exposing the body to cold water, you can activate specific neurochemical changes that improve mood, focus, and resilience.

Dopamine Surge

Cold exposure triggers a surge in dopamine, improving motivation, alertness, and overall mood.

Norepinephrine Release
Cold-water immersion boosts norepinephrine, a neurotransmitter that increases mental clarity and focus.

Serotonin and Endorphins
Regular cold exposure helps release serotonin and endorphins, contributing to a sense of well-being and pain relief.

Reduced Inflammation
Cold-water immersion reduces inflammation, benefiting recovery and reducing soreness, especially after intense physical activity.

Integrating Hydration and Cold Therapy for Optimal Health

Combining proper hydration with cold therapy can yield significant mental and physical benefits such as:

Better Mood
Regular hydration and cold exposure maintain healthy dopamine and serotonin levels, improving mood stability.

Enhanced Recovery
Cold therapy helps muscles recover faster and reduces inflammation, while hydration supports detoxification and muscle function.

Improved Focus and Clarity
Hydration and cold-water immersion enhance mental clarity by supporting optimal neurotransmitter levels.

Practical Tips for Hydration and Cold Therapy

Start Your Day Hydrated
Begin your morning with a glass of room-temperature water, possibly infused with lime or mint to support digestion and refresh the body.

Set Reminders for Hydration
Use reminders to prompt regular water intake throughout the day, especially during physical activity or in warm weather.

Incorporate Cold Therapy Gradually
Start with brief cold showers and slowly increase the duration. For those near bodies of water, consider short ocean plunges or cold baths.

Listen to Your Body
While cold therapy has many benefits, it's essential to approach it gradually and mindfully, especially if you have pre-existing conditions like heart disease.

Conclusion: Hydration and Cold Therapy for Longevity

Water is the foundation of health, supporting every system in the body, while cold therapy acts as a biohack to enhance neurotransmitter function and improve resilience. Whether it's through Ayurvedic hydration practices or cold-water immersion, these techniques offer simple yet powerful ways to optimize physical health, boost mental clarity, and promote emotional balance. By prioritizing hydration and integrating cold therapy into your routine, you can support long-term wellness and vitality—both at work and in everyday life, just like Lauren.

CHAPTER 25

BREATHWORK

Leena, a 42-year-old accountant in the heart of a bustling city, was the picture of resilience. By day, she tackled demanding work projects, meeting deadlines and making high-stakes decisions with precision. By night, she transitioned to her role as a mother, managing school schedules, helping with homework, and tending to her family's needs. Life was a constant rush, a delicate balancing act that left little room for rest. Over time, the pressures of her dual roles began to take a toll, and Leena found herself feeling perpetually anxious and mentally exhausted.

As the stress mounted, her body began sending her signals she couldn't ignore. Sleep became elusive, leaving her awake at odd hours, her mind racing. Digestive discomfort and unease settled in, symptoms she knew were signs of a deeper imbalance. Yet, despite her awareness, she couldn't find a way to break the cycle.

A close friend, noticing her struggle, suggested something unexpected—breathwork. Initially, Leena was skeptical. How could breathing, something she did every day without thinking, possibly help her find peace? But curiosity won out, and she decided to learn more. She consulted a local Ayurvedic practitioner who explained that her symptoms were likely rooted in a Vata imbalance. Together, they explored pranayama techniques designed to soothe her overstimulated energy and recalibrate her mental state.

With guidance, Leena began incorporating these breathwork practices into her daily routine. She learned to slow her breathing, anchoring her mind and calming her body. Gradually, she felt a subtle shift; her anxious thoughts began to quiet, and a sense of calm replaced the constant whirlwind in her mind. Nights brought restful sleep, her digestion improved, and, for the first time in a long while, she felt truly present—both at work and with her family. Breath by breath, Leena was reclaiming a balance she had long thought impossible.

Understanding Leena's Vata Imbalance

Leena's Ayurvedic consultation revealed that she was Vata-dominant. Vata dosha, governed by air and space, is associated with quick movement, changeability, and anxiety.

> **The practitioner noted that Leena's racing thoughts, restless mind, and irregular sleep patterns were typical signs of excess Vata.**

They explained that certain pranayama techniques could help calm her nervous system, lower anxiety, and stabilize dopamine and GABA levels—essential for mental clarity and emotional balance.

Leena's Tailored Breathwork Routine

The Ayurvedic practitioner recommended simple, calming breathwork exercises that could easily be integrated into Leena's daily routine.

Nadi Shodhana (Alternate-Nostril Breathing)

Leena was guided to sit comfortably, close her right nostril with her thumb, and inhale deeply through her left nostril. She then closed her left nostril with her ring finger and released her right nostril to exhale slowly.

This pattern was alternated for 10 minutes each morning and evening. Within a week, Leena noticed less mental agitation and a subtle calmness in her mind.

Sukh Pranayama (Gentle Breathing)

Leena added Sukh Pranayama to her morning routine, focusing on deep inhalations and longer exhalations, which stimulate GABA production.

Practicing this for 5 minutes each morning helped Leena start her day feeling grounded and clear-headed, setting a calmer tone for her busy workdays.

Aromatherapy with Lavender

To enhance her breathwork, Leena incorporated lavender essential oil, known for its calming effects. She diffused the oil during her evening sessions to create a more relaxing atmosphere.

This combination of aromatherapy and breathwork improved her ability to fall asleep and allowed her to wake up feeling more refreshed.

Diaphragmatic Breathing for Stress Reduction

Leena practiced diaphragmatic breathing during stressful moments at work. A general approach to diaphragmatic breathing includes:

- Find a Comfortable Position: Sit or lie down in a relaxed posture, ensuring your back is straight to facilitate optimal breathing.

- Place Your Hands: Position one hand on your chest and the other on your abdomen, just below the ribcage. This helps you monitor the movement of your diaphragm.

- Inhale Deeply Through the Nose: Breathe in slowly and deeply through your nose, allowing your abdomen to rise as the diaphragm contracts. Your chest should remain relatively still.

- Exhale Slowly Through the Mouth: Exhale gently through your mouth, feeling your abdomen fall as the diaphragm relaxes. Again, the chest should have minimal movement.

- Repeat the Process: Continue this pattern for several minutes, focusing on the rise and fall of your abdomen to ensure deep, diaphragmatic breaths.

Doing diaphragmatic breathing activated Leena's parasympathetic nervous system, reduced cortisol levels, and enabled her to respond more calmly to challenging situations.

Results of Leena's Breathwork Practice

After a month of consistent practice, Leena experienced several positive changes:

Reduced Anxiety

Nadi Shodhana and Sukh Pranayama helped lower her anxiety levels, making her feel more centered and less reactive to stress.

Improved Focus

Stimulating dopamine through rhythmic breathing increased her mental clarity, allowing her to concentrate for longer periods without feeling fatigued.

Better Sleep

Combining lavender aromatherapy with her evening breathwork improved her sleep quality and reduced nighttime restlessness.

Enhanced Digestion

Calming her Vata energy through deep breathing positively impacted her digestion, reducing bloating and discomfort.

Breathwork and Neurotransmitters: The Science of Calm

> **Breathing is more than just a way to supply oxygen to the body; it is a powerful tool for regulating the nervous system and influencing the brain's neurotransmitters, which in turn affect mood, stress levels, and cognitive function.**

Conscious, deep breathing helps activate the parasympathetic nervous system, which promotes rest and recovery. Here's how breathing affects neurotransmitters:

Dopamine

Rhythmic breathing patterns, such as those in Nadi Shodhana, can stimulate dopamine production, improving mental clarity, motivation, and emotional resilience.

GABA (Gamma-Aminobutyric Acid)

Slow, controlled breathing increases GABA production, making techniques like Sukh Pranayama particularly effective for reducing anxiety and calming the mind.

Serotonin

Deep breathing exercises boost serotonin levels, promoting mood stability and a sense of well-being. Serotonin is a precursor to melatonin, essential for regulating the sleep-wake cycle.

Cortisol

Breathwork reduces cortisol, the primary stress hormone, by activating the parasympathetic nervous system. Lower cortisol levels allow the body to recover from stress more effectively.

Pranayama: The Vedic Art of Breath Control

> **In the Vedic tradition, Pranayama involves controlled breathing techniques that regulate the flow of Prana (life force) throughout the body.**

It is central to yoga, Ayurveda, and meditation practices and is used to balance the doshas—Vata, Pitta, and Kapha. One of the most effective forms of pranayama for balancing Vata is Nadi Shodhana (alternate-nostril breathing), which harmonizes the energy flow between the brain's two hemispheres and creates a sense of inner peace.

How to Practice Nadi Shodhana

▌ Sit comfortably with your spine straight and shoulders relaxed.

▌ Close your right nostril with your thumb and inhale deeply through your left nostril.

▌ Close the left nostril with your ring finger, release the thumb from the right nostril, and exhale slowly.

▌ Inhale again through the right nostril, close it, and exhale through the left nostril.

▌ Continue alternating in this manner for several minutes.

This practice not only reduces stress but also helps balance Vata energy, which can become overstimulated in individuals prone to anxiety.

Nasal Cycles, Brain Hemispheres, and Breath

Scientific research has revealed that our breathing alternates between the right and left nostrils every 90 minutes, a phenomenon known as the nasal cycle. This cycle influences brain function: right-nostril breathing activates the left brain hemisphere, associated with logic and analytical tasks, while left-nostril breathing enhances the right brain hemisphere, linked to creativity and emotional processing.

Practicing alternate-nostril breathing can help create balance between the two brain hemispheres, leading to improved cognitive function and emotional stability.

Aromatherapy and Breathwork

> **Aromatherapy complements breathwork by stimulating the olfactory system, which directly influences the brain's emotional centers.**

Essential oils like lavender, eucalyptus, and peppermint enhance the calming or energizing effects of breathwork. For example, inhaling lavender oil before deep breathing can deepen relaxation and improve emotional well-being.

The Power of Breath for Mind, Body, and Spirit

Breathwork offers a simple yet profound tool for enhancing mental clarity, emotional resilience, and overall well-being. By consciously controlling the breath, you can balance neurotransmitters, calm the mind, and restore harmony to the doshas.

Whether practicing deep diaphragmatic breathing, Nadi Shodhana, or Sukh Pranayama, each technique has the potential to transform your mental and emotional state. Integrating breathwork into your daily routine—alongside Ayurvedic principles—can help you cultivate inner peace, improved focus, and long-term mental and physical health.

CHAPTER 26

YOGA ASANAS

Bill, a 39-year-old tech consultant, was known for his ambition and relentless work ethic. He thrived on the thrill of closing deals and navigating complex projects. But the intensity of his work was catching up with him. Day after day, he'd spend hours in front of his computer, battling tight deadlines, and it left him both mentally drained and physically tense. Despite his success, he found himself struggling with bouts of irritability, and even minor frustrations could set him off. He often felt overheated, as if his body were mirroring the pressure building inside him. Stress headaches became his constant companion, along with nagging digestive discomfort.

Determined to find relief, Bill decided to channel his energy into something new: yoga. Naturally competitive, he opted for a vigorous Power Yoga class, hoping that an intense workout would help him sweat out the tension. But after each session, Bill felt more restless than relaxed. The high-energy practice only seemed to fuel his irritability, leaving him overheated and struggling to unwind. It was as if he were pouring gasoline on the fire rather than calming it.

Frustrated, Bill realized he needed a different approach. Taking a step back, he decided to consult an Ayurvedic yoga instructor who could guide him toward something more in tune with his needs. The instructor quickly recognized Bill's pattern—a strong, fiery Pitta energy that was being aggravated by his lifestyle and his choice of intense exercise.

> **With a tailored plan, the instructor introduced Bill to cooling, grounding practices that would calm his mind and ease his tension, focusing on gentle asanas, calming breathwork, and relaxation techniques designed to balance his overactive Pitta.**

Gradually, Bill began to feel a shift. His headaches eased, his irritability softened, and his body felt less tense and overheated. For the first time in years, he found a sense of calm—not through pushing himself harder, but by finding balance within.

Understanding Bill's Pitta Imbalance

The instructor explained that Bill's primary dosha was Pitta, associated with the elements of fire and water. Pitta types often display intensity, focus, and ambition, but they are also prone to overheating and irritability, especially under stress. The instructor emphasized that Bill's yoga practice should focus on cooling, non-competitive, and calming postures to balance his Pitta energy.

Bill's Tailored Yoga Routine

The instructor designed a personalized yoga routine to cool Bill's Pitta, incorporating asanas, pranayama, and meditation. The practice was built around gentle movements and breath control, aiming to calm Bill's mind while cooling his body.

Cooling Yoga Postures

Bill's routine featured poses like Seated Forward Bend (Paschimottanasana). This pose, performed slowly, released physical tension and promoted mental calm, helping to reduce Pitta's heat and offering relief after a long workday.

Deep Breathing

Bill practiced diaphragmatic breathing to help regulate his body temperature and reduce feelings of irritation. The instructor encouraged Bill to use this technique whenever he felt frustrated at work, helping him stay composed in stressful situations.

Morning Meditation for Serotonin Balance

Bill incorporated a 15-minute morning meditation into his daily routine to stimulate serotonin production. This meditation helped Bill start his day calmly, setting a peaceful tone for work.

Evening Restorative Yoga

To unwind before bed, Bill practiced a short Restorative Yoga sequence. This routine helped him decompress and transition smoothly into sleep.

Results of Bill's Yoga Practice

Within a few months, Bill experienced noticeable improvements in both physical and mental well-being such as:

Reduced Irritability
Cooling and calming practices helped ease his irritability, enabling him to respond to stress with more patience.

Improved Focus
Balanced dopamine and serotonin levels enhanced his concentration, allowing him to complete tasks more effectively.

Better Sleep
Evening restorative poses and meditation improved sleep quality, allowing his body and mind to rejuvenate overnight.

Increased Emotional Stability
Bill felt more grounded and calm, with fewer mood swings and greater emotional balance.

Yoga and Neurotransmitters: Balancing the Brain

> **Yoga significantly impacts the brain's neurotransmitters, fostering an internal environment conducive to mental clarity, emotional balance, and focus.**

Dopamine
Physical movement and meditation increase dopamine levels, which enhance motivation, focus, and overall well-being. Studies show that yoga boosts dopamine release, helping with mood swings, attention deficits, and depression.

Serotonin

Deep breathing exercises (pranayama) and meditation stimulate serotonin production, helping to reduce anxiety and promote calmness.

GABA (Gamma-Aminobutyric Acid)

Styles like Hatha or Restorative Yoga significantly increase GABA levels, helping to relieve anxiety, PTSD, and ADHD. Even a single yoga session can lead to measurable increases in GABA, offering immediate stress relief.

Endorphins

Yoga postures, especially gentle stretching, trigger the release of endorphins, producing a sense of euphoria or a "yoga high." This is particularly helpful for managing chronic pain or emotional distress.

Brain-Derived Neurotrophic Factor (BDNF)

Yoga stimulates BDNF, a protein that promotes the growth and maintenance of neurons. This helps improve memory, learning, and protects the brain from age-related decline.

Yoga for the Doshas: Vata, Pitta, and Kapha

In Ayurveda, each dosha has distinct characteristics, and balancing these energies is essential for optimal health. Yoga can be personalized to suit each dosha's unique needs.

Yoga for Vata

Characteristics: Quick-thinking, energetic, but prone to anxiety and scattered thoughts.

Recommended Practices: Slow, grounding, and calming routines, such as Child's Pose (Balasana).

Focus: Emphasize stillness and stability, using gentle flows to prevent overstimulation.

Yoga for Pitta

Characteristics: Strong, focused, and driven, but prone to irritability and overheating.

Recommended Practices: Cooling, non-competitive yoga, including poses like Seated Forward Bend.

Focus: Don't overdue it especially with practices like hot yoga.

Yoga for Kapha

Characteristics: Calm, grounded, but prone to lethargy and emotional stagnation.

Recommended Practices: Stimulating, energizing routines with poses like Sun Salutations (Surya Namaskar).

Focus: Aim for dynamic, vigorous practices to increase energy and prevent stagnation.

Yoga as a Path to Balance and Well-Being

Yoga is not only a physical practice; it is a holistic approach that nurtures mental clarity, emotional balance, and spiritual growth.

By stimulating dopamine, serotonin, GABA, and BDNF, yoga creates a chemical environment in the brain that fosters long-term well-being.

For Bill, shifting from a competitive Power Yoga practice to a cooling and restorative routine helped reduce irritability, improve focus, and enhance emotional stability. By aligning his practice with his Pitta constitution, he discovered a path to sustainable balance.

Yoga, when tailored to an individual's unique dosha, can become a powerful tool for achieving mental clarity, emotional balance, and physical vitality. Whether you are a beginner or an experienced practitioner, integrating Ayurvedic principles into your practice can maximize yoga's benefits and help you achieve holistic health.

CHAPTER 27

MEDITATION

Ethan, a corporate lawyer at a high-stakes New York City firm, was the epitome of success—or so it seemed from the outside. His days were a blur of tight deadlines, complex cases, and relentless demands for peak performance. To keep up, Ethan leaned heavily on caffeine, fueling his early mornings and late nights with strong coffee, hoping it would sharpen his focus and keep his energy levels up. But no matter how much he drank, the stress only intensified, sinking deeper into his system and chipping away at his well-being.

At first, Ethan brushed off the signs. He told himself that the fatigue, restlessness, and irritability were just part of the job, a price he was willing to pay for success. Yet his sleep grew increasingly erratic; he'd lie awake in the early hours, mind spinning with worries about cases, and his mood swings became harder to ignore.

One evening, after a particularly grueling day in the office, Ethan felt his chest tighten, his breath catching as anxiety washed over him. His heart raced, and his hands grew clammy. In that moment, he feared he might be on the verge of a breakdown. It was a wake-up call he couldn't ignore. This wasn't just a bad day; his body was warning him that he couldn't keep pushing himself like this.

As he calmed down, Ethan knew something had to change. He realized that his health and sanity were worth more than any deadline, and he was finally ready to explore a new path—a path that would allow him to take back control of his life, reduce his stress, and reclaim his well-being.

Ethan's Introduction to Transcendental Meditation (TM)

A colleague noticed Ethan's struggles and suggested he try Transcendental Meditation (TM), a practice that had helped her manage work stress. Initially skeptical, Ethan decided to give it a shot. He enrolled in a TM course, which included personal instruction and follow-up sessions to ensure he could practice effectively.

Ethan found TM surprisingly simple.

> **Unlike other forms of meditation he had tried, TM required no focus or effort to control thoughts. It involved a specific technique that allowed the mind to naturally settle into a state of restful awareness.**

Within just a week of practicing TM twice daily for 20 minutes, Ethan noticed a significant reduction in anxiety and a quieter mental state.

Meditation's Impact on Ethan's Neurotransmitter Balance

As Ethan continued with TM, he experienced deeper benefits:

Serotonin Increase: Ethan felt more emotionally balanced and less reactive to stress.

Cortisol Reduction: Ethan's stress hormone levels dropped, reflected in lower blood pressure and improved sleep.

Practicing TM in the morning helped Ethan start his day with mental clarity, while an evening session allowed him to unwind and sleep more soundly. Meditation also improved his neuroadaptability, enabling him to bounce back quickly from stressful events.

Ethan's Transformation

Six months into his TM routine, Ethan's life had transformed:

Better Focus and Productivity
With increased dopamine levels, Ethan felt sharper and more engaged during meetings and client interactions.

Improved Relationships
Colleagues noted his newfound patience, and Ethan felt more present with family.

Improved Health
Numerous studies have shown how TM can reduce blood pressure. When Ethan went to his doctor he was happy to see his blood pressure had dropped into a healthy range again.

TM also balanced Ethan's Pitta dosha, reducing his intense focus, and irritability. Meditation helped "cool" his mind, promoting a more adaptable and harmonious approach to work and personal life.

Meditation: An Antidote to Modern Stress

Stress is the underlying cause of many physical and mental health issues, including anxiety, heart disease, and depression. It also drives unhealthy habits like smoking and overeating, creating a vicious cycle. Meditation offers a way to break this cycle, restore balance, and support both body and mind.

The Neuroscience of Meditation: How It Influences Neurotransmitters

> **Transcendental Meditation creates a state of restful alertness, marked by increased alpha brain waves in the prefrontal cortex, a region involved in decision-making, emotional regulation, and focus. It also positively affects several key neurotransmitters:**

Dopamine
Increases during meditation, enhancing focus, motivation, and also mood.

Serotonin
Levels rise, reducing anxiety and promoting emotional stability.

GABA
Deep relaxation techniques boost GABA, leading to calmness and well-being.

Endorphins
Meditation triggers endorphin release, improving mood and reducing stress.

Cortisol
Meditation reduces cortisol, the primary stress hormone, reversing the damage caused by chronic stress.

Stress, Dopamine, and the Fight-or-Flight Response

Stress activates the brain's fight-or-flight response, driven by the amygdala. In stressful situations, cortisol and adrenaline levels surge, preparing the body to either fight or flee. While this response is helpful in immediate danger, its chronic activation—as seen in today's fast-paced life—depletes dopamine, contributing to fatigue, lack of motivation, and depression.

Regular meditation calms the amygdala, reducing cortisol production and restoring dopamine balance. This helps the brain transition from a reactive to a responsive state, promoting better mental health and resilience.

Types of Meditation: Understanding the Differences

Meditation practices can be categorized into three main types based on how they influence the brain:

Focused Attention
Involves concentrating on a single object, like the breath or a mantra. Increases gamma brain waves (20-50 Hz), associated with intense focus.

Open Monitoring

Observes thoughts and feelings without judgment. Increases theta brain waves (4-8 Hz), linked to creativity and relaxed awareness.

Automatic Self-Transcending

TM falls into this category, allowing the mind to naturally transcend mental activity. Increases alpha brain waves (8-10 Hz), associated with deep relaxation and coherent brain activity.

TM stands out because it doesn't require focus or control. It allows the mind to settle effortlessly, balancing neurotransmitters like dopamine and serotonin, creating a sense of calm, clarity, and inner peace.

Meditation and Neuroadaptability: Building Resilience

> **Neuroadaptability is the brain's ability to adapt to and recover from stress.**

Chronic stress weakens this adaptability, making individuals more prone to anxiety, depression, and cognitive decline. TM strengthens neuroadaptability by enhancing communication between the prefrontal cortex and amygdala, the brain's emotional centers.

Studies show that regular TM practice increases alpha wave coherence, improving emotional regulation, decision-making, and creativity. This means that individuals like Ethan can respond to stress more effectively, maintaining mental balance even under pressure.

Research on Transcendental Meditation and Health

Over 600 studies conducted at more than 200 research institutions have documented Transcendental Meditation's benefits (see Appendix 3). Highlights include:

Cardiovascular Health
A study funded by the National Institutes of Health (NIH) found a 48% reduction in heart attacks, strokes, and deaths among TM practitioners compared to non-meditators.

Reduced Aging
Long-term TM practitioners have younger biological ages and longer telomeres, suggesting slowed cellular aging.

Improved Mental Health
Research shows significant reductions in anxiety, depression, and PTSD among TM practitioners.

Ayurveda and Meditation: Balancing the Doshas

Meditation is central to Ayurveda's approach to balancing the doshas—Vata, Pitta, and Kapha:

Vata
Prone to anxiety and scattered thoughts. Meditation calms and grounds Vata energy.

Pitta

Prone to anger, irritability, and perfectionism. Meditation cools Pitta's intensity, promoting patience and compassion.

Kapha

Prone to lethargy and resistance to change. Meditation energizes and prevents stagnation.

The Power of Meditation for Stress Relief and Longevity

Meditation, particularly TM, is a powerful tool for reducing stress, balancing neurotransmitters, and enhancing mental clarity. By incorporating regular meditation into daily life, you can cultivate inner peace, resilience, and adaptability—no matter how demanding your environment. Ethan's story is a testament to the transformative power of meditation, showing that it's not just a tool for managing stress but a path to mental, emotional, and physical well-being.

CHAPTER 28

HAPPINESS

Rachel, a 58-year-old art teacher in Los Angeles, was known for her vibrant personality and her ability to bring out the creative spark in her students. Her life had always been filled with color and emotion, whether in her own artwork, in her classroom, or in the memories of raising her children. Art had given her purpose, and being a mother had filled her days with love. But as her children grew older and moved on to build lives of their own, a quiet emptiness began to settle in—a feeling Rachel hadn't anticipated.

At first, she tried to ignore it, pouring herself into her teaching and her painting. But no matter how many canvases she filled or classes she taught, something felt off. The house felt too quiet, her heart a bit too heavy. Rachel realized she was struggling with a loneliness she couldn't paint away. Her days, once brimming with laughter and purpose, felt a little dimmer, and her joy seemed to slip further from her grasp.

Curious and determined to understand her emotions better, Rachel began exploring the science behind happiness. She discovered how deeply neurotransmitters like dopamine, serotonin, oxytocin, and endorphins could influence feelings of joy, connection, and fulfillment. Intrigued, she decided to try a new approach, weaving daily habits into her routine that could naturally boost these "happiness chemicals."

Rachel started with small steps. She took long walks in nature to lift her serotonin, practiced gratitude each morning to nurture her endorphins, and reached out to old friends, sparking her oxytocin. She even joined a local art class, finding inspiration and joy in the camaraderie of fellow artists. Slowly, Rachel felt her world brightening. The same creative spirit that had once filled her life now held new meaning, guiding her back to a sense of purpose.

With each passing day, Rachel found herself rediscovering joy—not only through her art and teaching but in the simple moments of connection and self-care.

> **Her journey became a beautiful reminder that happiness, like art, is something we can create, layer by layer, even when the colors of life begin to change.**

Implementing Ayurvedic Behavioral Rasayanas

Rachel's first step was to explore Ayurveda's behavioral rasayanas, practices designed to rejuvenate body and mind:

Creating a Stable Routine
Rachel set regular meal times, embraced a consistent bedtime, and began meditating daily. This structure helped calm her Vata dosha, which had been contributing to her restless thoughts.

Acts of Kindness

Rachel also made a point of engaging in small, kind gestures—whether complimenting a colleague, smiling at a stranger, or supporting a friend. These simple acts brought her immediate feelings of warmth, boosting oxytocin, the "love hormone" linked to compassion and connectedness.

Reconnecting with Relationships

Recognizing that strong social bonds are essential for happiness, Rachel reached out to old friends for coffee dates and made it a point to visit her children more frequently. She also began hosting monthly art nights, inviting neighbors and colleagues for an evening of painting and laughter. These gatherings lifted her mood and gave her a sense of purpose, creating more social interaction and fostering community.

Finding Joy through Creativity

Art had always been Rachel's passion, but she now committed to painting daily, turning it into a therapeutic ritual. This practice not only helped her express emotions but also stimulated dopamine release, bringing a renewed sense of motivation. As she immersed herself in creative flow, she found a deep sense of fulfillment and accomplishment.

Meditation for Inner Peace

Rachel also deepened her meditation practice, dedicating twenty minutes each morning to meditation and focused breathing. As the weeks passed, she felt calmer and more content, a result of increased serotonin and GABA. Meditation also helped lower her cortisol levels, improving her sleep quality and emotional balance.

Rekindling Purpose

Rachel's happiness blossomed as she discovered a new purpose: teaching a weekend art class for senior citizens. Sharing the therapeutic benefits of art brought Rachel immense joy, as she watched her students express themselves creatively and build friendships. This new venture not only filled her heart but also gave her a renewed sense of mission.

> **Rachel's consistent efforts—nurturing neurotransmitters, building relationships, and pursuing creative activities—led to a profound transformation. Her happiness wasn't just about fleeting pleasure; it became a deep, lasting sense of fulfillment.**

The Biology of Happiness: Understanding Neurotransmitters

Happiness plays a vital role in health and longevity. Studies show that happier people experience:

- Better immune function

- Lower blood pressure

- Reduced risk of heart disease

- Greater mental well-being

But how do neurotransmitters like dopamine, serotonin, oxytocin, and endorphins contribute to happiness?

Dopamine: The Motivator

Dopamine drives anticipation and motivation more than actual pleasure. It is the "wanting" neurotransmitter, urging us to pursue rewards like food, social media, or addictive behaviors. While it's vital for motivation, an over-reliance on dopamine can create a cycle of diminishing returns, as the brain reduces its sensitivity, requiring more stimulation for the same level of pleasure.

Serotonin: The Stabilizer

Serotonin is associated with contentment and emotional stability. High serotonin levels foster feelings of peace, well-being, and satisfaction. Activities like meditation, sunlight exposure, and exercise naturally boost serotonin, promoting longer-lasting happiness.

Oxytocin: The Connection Hormone

Released during moments of affection and connection, oxytocin fosters warmth, trust, and love. It is essential for forming bonds and feeling a sense of belonging. Higher oxytocin levels are linked to increased happiness and social connections.

Endorphins: The Natural Painkillers

Endorphins contribute to euphoria and stress relief, helping us manage discomfort while maintaining a positive outlook. Endorphins are released during exercise, laughter, and even creative activities, making them essential for emotional resilience.

Happiness and Relationships: The Role of Social Bonds

Strong relationships are among the strongest predictors of happiness and longevity. Research on populations in Blue

Zones—regions with high concentrations of centenarians—shows that social bonds and supportive relationships are key to physical and mental well-being.

> **Relationships not only enhance immune function and reduce stress, but they also provide a sense of purpose and connection.**

Conversely, loneliness has been linked to increased inflammation, weakened immunity, and a higher risk of addiction.

Ayurveda and Happiness

Ayurveda offers holistic ways to nurture happiness through these behavioral rasayanas:

- Balanced Routine: Stability helps calm Vata and creates a foundation for peace.

- Acts of Kindness: Compassionate acts release oxytocin, strengthening social bonds and emotional well-being.

- Positive Communication: Speaking truthfully and kindly fosters harmony and reduces emotional stress.

- Patience and Equanimity: Reducing anger and frustration helps balance Pitta and maintain inner peace.

- Higher Consciousness: Meditation fosters transcendence, balancing dopamine, serotonin, and GABA for sustained happiness.

Purpose and Creativity: Keys to Lasting Joy

Engaging in creativity and finding purpose are essential to happiness. Studies show that older adults who engage in creative pursuits like painting, music, or writing experience greater well-being and life satisfaction.

Purpose is equally important. Whether it's caring for family, volunteering, or pursuing personal goals, having a sense of purpose fosters emotional fulfillment and resilience against challenges. Rachel's commitment to teaching art to seniors exemplifies how purpose can reignite happiness and provide a sense of mission.

True Happiness: A Journey, Not Just a Feeling

Happiness is more than fleeting pleasure; it is about creating balance, nurturing relationships, and pursuing meaningful goals. While dopamine drives us to seek rewards, serotonin, oxytocin, and endorphins create deeper joy. By incorporating Ayurvedic practices like behavioral rasayanas, fostering social bonds, and pursuing creative and purposeful activities, we can cultivate true, long-lasting happiness.

Rachel's story is a testament to the idea that happiness is not just an emotion—it is a practice that enhances both mind and body. By building relationships, engaging in creative pursuits, and finding purpose, Rachel rediscovered her joy. Her journey shows that happiness is within reach, even in life's later stages. With intention and effort, we can all cultivate a life of fulfillment and joy.

CHAPTER 29

SOCIAL INTERACTIONS

David, a 43-year-old engineer with a relentless work ethic, and Priya, a 40-year-old yoga instructor with a calm and gentle approach to life, had shared a deep bond for over 12 years. Their marriage had always been rooted in love, trust, and a shared respect for one another's values. Their differences, once a source of balance, seemed to make them stronger. David's Pitta-driven ambition and determination brought structure to their lives, while Priya's Kapha-nurturing spirit provided warmth and stability. They complemented each other perfectly—or so it seemed in the early years.

But as time passed, those once-harmonious differences began to wear on them. David's high-energy approach to life, fueled by his drive to excel in his career, often clashed with Priya's slower-paced, reflective lifestyle. David found himself feeling increasingly frustrated by Priya's tendency to resist change, perceiving her grounded nature as stagnation. Meanwhile, Priya felt overwhelmed and even exhausted by David's intensity, yearning for a gentler rhythm that honored her need for peace and connection.

The tension between them grew, slowly building walls that neither of them wanted but couldn't quite break down. Their conversations turned into debates, their quiet evenings into silent retreats into separate corners of the house. They both felt the distance growing, and it hurt to see the closeness they had once cherished slipping away.

One evening, after a particularly tense exchange, Priya took a deep breath and suggested something different. "What if we tried approaching this from an Ayurvedic perspective?" she asked, a spark of hope in her eyes. Priya had seen Ayurveda transform her own life and the lives of her yoga students, and she wondered if its wisdom could help bridge the gap between them. David, though usually a skeptic of alternative approaches, found himself intrigued by Ayurveda's logical approach and data-backed insights into human nature. He agreed to explore how understanding their doshas—Pitta and Kapha—might help them reconnect.

Together, they embarked on a journey of self-discovery. They learned how David's Pitta, with its fiery drive, could sometimes overpower Priya's Kapha, which thrived on steadiness and patience. They discovered ways to balance their energies: David practiced slowing down and appreciating stillness, while Priya embraced small, manageable changes that brought variety into her routine without overwhelming her. They introduced shared rituals into their daily life, from evening walks to moments of mindfulness, giving each other the space to be themselves while finding common ground.

As they embraced Ayurveda's teachings, they began to see each other with fresh eyes. David learned to appreciate Priya's grounding presence as a source of calm amidst his busy world, and Priya found admiration for David's drive, recognizing it as an expression of passion rather than intensity. Slowly, the walls between them faded, replaced by a renewed respect and a deeper understanding of each other.

In their journey, they discovered that true love isn't just about shared values; it's also about learning to navigate and honor each other's differences.

> **Through Ayurveda, David and Priya rekindled not only their connection but also a newfound appreciation for the dance between their contrasting energies—a dance that would keep their relationship vibrant for years to come.**

Implementing Ayurvedic Insights for Relationship Harmony

David and Priya began to apply Ayurvedic principles to balance their individual energies and deepen their bond.

Balancing Pitta and Kapha
David recognized that his intense approach often led to impatience. He learned that Priya, as a Kapha, needed more time to adapt to new ideas. By adjusting his communication style—slowing down and allowing Priya space to respond—David found that conflicts became less frequent.

Cooling Down Pitta's Fire
David integrated cooling practices into his routine, like evening meditation and calming yoga poses. These practices helped him manage his intensity, enabling more empathetic interactions with Priya.

Energizing Kapha

Priya was encouraged to engage in more dynamic activities to stimulate her energy. The couple began taking morning runs or dance classes together, helping Priya break free from lethargy while creating shared moments of joy.

Regular Meals and Routines

Ayurveda emphasizes regular meal times, especially in Pitta-Kapha relationships. David and Priya made it a point to eat together consistently, strengthening their sense of routine, connection, and balance.

Oxytocin through Physical Touch

They consciously added more physical touch—longer hugs, holding hands, and warm embraces—into their daily interactions. This simple act boosted oxytocin, fostering warmth, security, and deeper intimacy.

Rediscovering Connection Through Neurotransmitters

In addition to Ayurveda's dosha-balancing practices, David and Priya explored the role of neurotransmitters in their relationship.

Dopamine and Excitement

To revive the spark in their relationship, they planned spontaneous date nights and weekend getaways. These dopamine-boosting experiences rekindled excitement and motivation, bringing back the thrill they felt when they first met.

Serotonin and Stability

The couple began morning walks in the sunlight and practiced daily gratitude exercises. These habits boosted serotonin, which enhanced their emotional stability and helped manage conflicts with greater patience.

Oxytocin and Bonding

They set aside time for deep conversations—sharing feelings, dreams, and fears without judgment. This increased their sense of trust, security, and emotional closeness, reinforcing oxytocin and deepening their bond.

A Renewed Relationship

> **With Ayurvedic guidance and a focus on neurotransmitter balance, David and Priya discovered a new way to align their energies and create harmony.**

David learned to temper his Pitta-driven impatience, while Priya found the motivation to embrace change and new activities. Their commitment to understanding each other's doshas, along with the influence of neurotransmitters on their interactions, fostered a balanced and fulfilling relationship.

David and Priya's story illustrates that harmonious relationships require conscious effort, patience, and a genuine willingness to understand each other's needs. By integrating Ayurveda's wisdom and neurochemical insights, they not only healed their relationship but also enhanced their overall well-being.

Relationships and Well-being: The Ayurvedic Perspective

Relationships profoundly impact our emotional and physical health, shaping both happiness and well-being. Ayurveda offers valuable insights into how we can nurture relationships, using the understanding of doshas and neurotransmitters to create harmony.

The Role of Neurotransmitters in Relationships

> **Neurotransmitters—dopamine, serotonin, oxytocin, and endorphins—play pivotal roles in shaping our emotional bonds.**

Dopamine
This neurotransmitter is released during moments of excitement and reward, driving attraction and motivation in the early stages of relationships. It also reinforces positive behaviors, contributing to lasting bonds.

Serotonin
In relationships, serotonin promotes emotional stability and contentment. It helps partners maintain patience, manage conflicts empathetically, and foster a deeper sense of trust.

Oxytocin
Oxytocin is released during moments of physical intimacy and emotional connection. It fosters closeness, trust, and security, playing a crucial role in both romantic and parental bonds.

Endorphins
These natural painkillers create positive feelings and reduce stress during shared activities, helping partners experience joy and resilience in the relationship.

Ayurveda's Dosha-Based Compatibility in Relationships

Ayurveda emphasizes the importance of understanding each person's dosha balance in relationships. Each combination of doshas brings unique dynamics and challenges.

Vata Partner / Vata Partner
Strengths: Creativity, enthusiasm, and a love for new experiences.
Challenges: Prone to emotional swings, misunderstandings, and hypersensitivity.
Advice: Establish grounding routines and engage in calming activities like gentle yoga or meditation.

Pitta Partner / Pitta Partner
Strengths: Passion, energy, and ambition.
Challenges: Heated arguments, competitiveness, and controlling behaviors.
Advice: Focus on maintaining a cool, calm environment, support stress reduction, and channel energy positively.

Kapha Partner / Kapha Partner
Strengths: Steadiness, reliability, and nurturing.
Challenges: Stagnation, lethargy, and emotional withdrawal.
Advice: Engage in stimulating activities together, maintain social interactions, and encourage each other to stay active.

Vata Partner / Pitta Partner

Strengths: Dynamic, with Vata's creativity complementing Pitta's drive.

Challenges: Volatility due to Pitta's intensity and Vata's sensitivity.

Advice: Prioritize empathy, open communication, and balance through relaxation and shared routines.

Vata Partner / Kapha Partner

Strengths: Vata's spontaneity brings excitement, while Kapha provides stability.

Challenges: Vata may feel Kapha is too slow; Kapha may find Vata too erratic.

Advice: Appreciate differences, maintain a shared routine, and engage in activities that blend energy levels.

Pitta Partner / Kapha Partner

Strengths: Pitta's ambition complements Kapha's grounding nature.

Challenges: Pitta's impatience may clash with Kapha's inertia.

Advice: Pitta should slow down; Kapha should become more active. Balance can be achieved through regular meals, relaxing activities, and open communication.

The Intersection of Neurotransmitters and Doshas

Neurotransmitters align with dosha dynamics, shaping how partners experience connection:

> Dopamine enhances excitement and motivation, aligning well with Pitta's driven energy.

▌ Serotonin fosters emotional stability, crucial for Kapha's steady nature.

▌ Oxytocin strengthens bonds, creating the security and trust needed by Vata's sensitive temperament.

Cultivating Harmony in Relationships

Ayurveda's holistic approach, combined with an understanding of neurotransmitter influences, provides a roadmap for nurturing harmonious relationships. David and Priya's journey demonstrates that successful relationships require balance, presence, and a willingness to understand each other's needs. By consciously working to maintain dosha balance and neurochemical harmony, couples can foster deeper connections and enhance their mental and physical well-being.

CHAPTER 30

SPIRITUALITY

Sarah, a 51-year-old environmentalist and nature photographer, had spent decades chasing the untamed beauty of the natural world. Her life had been a tapestry of adventure, with each photograph capturing breathtaking landscapes and elusive wildlife. From misty mountains to tranquil forests, her work reflected a profound love for the earth—a love she hoped would inspire others to protect its fragile wonders.

Yet, as fulfilling as her work was, Sarah felt an ache growing within her, a sense of emptiness that lingered in the quiet moments. Her children, once the center of her universe, had grown up and moved on to start families of their own. The once-busy home was now silent, its rooms filled only with echoes of laughter and memories. Her outdoor adventures, once shared with them, now seemed bittersweet, reminding her of their absence.

She threw herself into her photography, hoping it would fill the void. But each shot, each journey, brought only a fleeting sense of joy. She could capture the grandeur of a sunrise or the delicate beauty of a wildflower, yet the fulfillment she sought remained elusive, slipping through her fingers like sand.

One evening, sitting alone in her studio and scrolling through photos of her latest trip, Sarah realized what she was truly missing.

She had always seen her art as a way to connect others to nature, but what she longed for now was a deeper connection herself—a purpose that extended beyond images and adventures, something that could bring her a sense of belonging and contribution beyond her role as a photographer.

Determined to find new meaning, Sarah began exploring ways to use her skills to educate others about environmental conservation. She started hosting photography workshops for young nature enthusiasts and volunteering to document local conservation efforts, lending her lens to causes that would benefit from her perspective. She even considered turning her work into a book, not just as a collection of images, but as a guide to inspire others to see the earth with fresh eyes and open hearts.

> **As Sarah's efforts expanded, so did her sense of purpose. She realized that her life's work was no longer just about capturing nature's beauty—it was about giving back, creating a legacy that would nurture the love she held for the planet in others.**

With each workshop, each conservation project, she found the emptiness slowly fading, replaced by a quiet joy that rooted her as deeply as the forests she loved to photograph. Her purpose, she discovered, was still alive and evolving, blossoming like a wildflower in the light of her own rediscovered passion.

Searching for Deeper Meaning

Sarah realized that she needed more than temporary highs

from her work or hobbies; she sought a deeper connection with life. Curious about the science of spirituality and its impact on neurotransmitters like dopamine and serotonin, she decided to explore Ayurveda and meditation to find a sense of peace and fulfillment.

Integrating Ayurveda and Spiritual Practices

Sarah began her spiritual journey with a holistic approach rooted in Ayurveda, which emphasizes the mind-body-spirit connection. Her Ayurvedic practitioner identified Vata imbalance as a source of her restlessness, explaining that grounding spiritual practices could help stabilize her emotions and restore a sense of peace.

Here's how Sarah incorporated spirituality into her life:

Meditation for Dopamine and Serotonin Balance
Sarah started practicing Transcendental Meditation (TM) twice daily. This effortless technique increased motivation and joy, while also boosting serotonin, promoting inner peace. Over time, meditation transformed her sense of happiness from fleeting highs to a stable, enduring state of contentment.

Connecting with Nature for Oxytocin and Unity
Already an avid hiker, Sarah began to engage with nature more mindfully. She listened to the sounds of birds, felt the textures of leaves, and breathed in the earthy scent of the forest. This conscious connection to nature increased oxytocin, fostering a sense of unity with the environment. Her hikes became more than physical activities; they became sacred moments of spiritual communion.

Vedic Sound Therapy for Coherence and Inner Stillness

Sarah added Vedic Sound Therapy to her routine, listening to specific mantras that were recommended with her. These sounds created coherent brainwave patterns, which improved mental clarity and deepened her spiritual connection. She described the effect as an "experience of oneness," a feeling of merging with a larger, universal consciousness.

Daily Gratitude as a Spiritual Practice

Sarah incorporated a daily gratitude ritual, acknowledging both small and big blessings. This simple practice increased her serotonin levels, fostering a sense of contentment. Gratitude became a spiritual exercise that aligned her thoughts with positive beliefs, reinforcing feelings of happiness and fulfillment.

Transforming Through Spirituality

Sarah's commitment to spiritual practices gradually shifted her entire outlook.

She discovered a renewed sense of purpose, not just in her work, but in her everyday existence. She began to see her nature photography as an act of spiritual expression, a way of capturing the divine beauty of the world.

Her spiritual journey fostered profound inner peace and joy, improving her relationships with others. Sarah became more compassionate, patient, and open, qualities that reflected oxytocin's influence. The newfound sense of calm and clarity made her more resilient to challenges, helping her maintain balance across her mind, body, and spirit.

The Neuroscience of Sarah's Transformation

Sarah's spiritual practices created lasting changes in her brain chemistry:

I Dopamine fueled her motivation to explore spirituality, providing joy and anticipation as she embraced new practices.

I Serotonin brought emotional stability, allowing her to achieve a calm, contented state of mind.

I Oxytocin strengthened her sense of connection to nature, herself, and others, fostering trust and love.

I Endorphins contributed to well-being during meditation and nature walks, enhancing her overall happiness.

With spirituality now integrated into her daily routine, Sarah's sense of inner peace, joy, and purpose flourished. She continued her nature photography with a more profound perspective, seeing it not just as a career, but as a spiritual act of celebrating life's beauty. By aligning her mind, body, and spirit with the rhythms of nature, Sarah found the fulfillment that had once seemed beyond reach.

The Neuroscience of Spirituality

Spiritual experiences—whether through meditation, prayer, or immersion in nature—are often accompanied by shifts in brain chemistry.

Dopamine

Meaningful spiritual practices stimulate dopamine pathways, leading to feelings of joy and motivation. This explains why engaging in spirituality can be as rewarding as physical or material pleasures.

Serotonin

Practices like meditation or prayer increase serotonin, which contributes to emotional peace and satisfaction.

Oxytocin

Rituals and shared spiritual beliefs release oxytocin, fostering a sense of belonging and connection. This chemical plays a key role in creating strong social bonds within spiritual communities.

Endorphins

Spiritual activities, including rituals, music, and dancing, release endorphins, promoting feelings of euphoria and emotional resilience.

The Placebo Effect and the Power of Belief

The intersection of spirituality and neuroscience is perhaps best illustrated by the placebo effect, where the mind's belief in healing triggers real physical changes. Neuroimaging studies reveal that meditation and spirituality can stimulate neurotransmitters like dopamine and endorphins, reducing pain and improving mood.

Dr. Alia Crum's research at Stanford University shows that positive beliefs can alter physiological responses, highlighting the mind's profound impact on health. Her studies suggest that spiritual beliefs and practices may act as powerful placebos, fostering health through hope, faith, and positive thinking.

Spirituality and Consciousness in Ayurveda

Ayurveda sees spirituality as essential for balancing the doshas—Vata, Pitta, and Kapha. Spiritual growth is not just about mental clarity but about cultivating a deeper connection to universal energy, or pure consciousness.

> **In his book *Consciousness Is All There Is*, Dr. Tony Nader emphasizes how meditation and spiritual practices promote coherent brainwave patterns, leading to refined nervous system functioning and higher states of consciousness.**

Research suggests that spiritual experiences can awaken a new level of awareness, where individuals perceive a seamless connection between themselves and nature.

Finding Fulfillment through Spirituality

Sarah's journey is a testament to spirituality's power to transform life. By integrating spiritual practices—meditation, nature immersion, Vedic Sound Therapy, and gratitude—into daily routines, one can achieve lasting fulfillment. Spirituality, as Ayurveda teaches, fosters balance, peace, and a sense of unity with all of life.

Spiritual growth is not just about fleeting happiness; it's about cultivating inner stillness, neurochemical balance, and a pro-found sense of purpose. By embracing spiritual practices, we can transcend the limitations of ordinary experience, touching the infinite within and enhancing overall well-being.

.

CHAPTER 31

COLLECTIVE CONSCIOUSNESS

Carlos, a 65-year-old retired psychology professor, had spent his life nurturing the minds and spirits of those around him. In his small coastal town in California, he was known not only for his wisdom but for his warm, open heart. Whether he was leading a community workshop, helping to organize a local event, or volunteering with neighborhood groups, Carlos found joy in connecting with others. His days were rich with purpose, and he cherished the sense of belonging that came from being woven into the fabric of his community.

But when his wife passed away, everything changed. She had been his closest confidant, his partner in every way, and the love of his life. Without her, the world felt achingly quiet. The vibrant life he'd built seemed to lose its color, and even the bustling town he had once adored now seemed like a distant echo. The community gatherings he once loved felt hollow, the laughter and camaraderie a reminder of his own solitude. He attended fewer events, his days growing lonelier, filled with a longing for the connection he once took for granted.

Carlos knew he couldn't continue this way. He wanted to honor his wife's memory by returning to the world they had once shared, but he struggled to find his place without her by his side. After months of quiet reflection, he decided to start small. He began by volunteering at the town's senior center, offering counseling and support to others who, like him, were navigating the complexities of aging and loss. He started hosting weekly discussion groups, drawing on his experience as a psychologist to guide conversations on grief, resilience, and finding new purpose.

Gradually, Carlos found himself rekindling the connection he had lost. His groups became a lifeline not only for others but for himself. He was moved by the stories shared, the laughter that returned, and the friendships that began to form. And with each new connection, he felt his own heart healing.

In time, Carlos realized that he was creating something beautiful—a new community woven together by shared experiences and mutual support. His life, once filled with sorrow, was now filled with purpose again, each day an opportunity to bring comfort and strength to others. Through his efforts, he discovered that even in the face of profound loss, there was still a way forward, a path to joy that honored the love he had lost while embracing the life he still had.

Rediscovering Community and Collective Consciousness

> **Carlos joined a local Transcendental Meditation (TM) group that practiced together regularly. Through twice-daily group meditation, he experienced not only personal calm but also a stronger sense of unity with his community.**

The group's intention was to create peace and coherence throughout the town, inspired by the Maharishi Effect, which a number of researcher studies have shown that group meditation can positively influence the surrounding environment (see Appendix 4). This concept gave Carlos a renewed sense of purpose—his personal meditation practice was now a contribution to community well-being.

Intergenerational Activities for Social Bonding

Drawing from his background as an educator, Carlos initiated a "Wisdom Exchange" program at the local community center. Older adults, like Carlos, shared life stories, skills, and advice with younger participants.

These gatherings not only built bridges across generations but also increased oxytocin, fostering trust and connection. Carlos noticed significant improvements in his mood after each session, as the interactions boosted feel-good chemicals like serotonin and dopamine.

Creating Social Rituals for Connection

Inspired by Ayurvedic principles of social rituals, Carlos organized weekly community potluck dinners, where neighbors gathered to share food, laughter, and conversation.

These shared meals quickly became a cherished tradition, increasing oxytocin and serotonin, and fostering a sense of safety, belonging, and happiness within the community.

Encouraging Healthy Routines in the Community

Carlos collaborated with others to establish weekly walking

groups, sunrise yoga by the beach, and a monthly "day of service." These regular activities provided structure and purpose, while also promoting physical health and releasing dopamine.

Creating Spaces for Reflection and Meditation

Carlos spearheaded a project to create a community garden with a designated area for reflection and meditation. Open to all, this serene space allowed individuals to connect with nature and engage in meditation practices. Carlos found that spending time here boosted his serotonin levels and brought a sense of spiritual connection.

Carlos' Transformation Through Collective Consciousness

As Carlos re-engaged with his community through these practices, he noticed significant improvements in his mental and emotional well-being. His loneliness diminished, replaced by a sense of purpose and belonging. The regular meditation sessions, social gatherings, and communal activities not only lifted his mood but also restored his motivation and zest for life.

Carlos experienced firsthand how collective consciousness transformed his personal health:

- Dopamine increased through meaningful social interactions, improving his motivation and emotional resilience.

- Serotonin rose as he found contentment and stability through regular social rituals and meditation.

- Oxytocin surged during moments of physical and emotional closeness, fostering deeper bonds and trust.

> Endorphins were released during group walks and exercise, contributing to a sense of well-being and reducing stress.

Carlos remains dedicated to fostering collective consciousness through regular group meditation, intergenerational programs, and shared rituals that promote peace, unity, and happiness. He has become a catalyst for community well-being, inspiring others to join him in creating a supportive and thriving environment.

The Power of Collective Consciousness in Ayurveda and Neuroscience

> **From the perspective of Ayurveda and neuroscience, community engagement and collective consciousness are integral to health and longevity.**

Social connections are closely tied to the regulation of neurotransmitters like dopamine, serotonin, oxytocin, and endorphins, which govern our mood, motivation, and sense of well-being.

Here are strategies to enhance collective consciousness:

Encourage Social Rituals
Regular social rituals like shared meals, festivals, or group meditation activate oxytocin and serotonin pathways, fostering a sense of belonging and emotional well-being.

Foster Intergenerational Connections
Intergenerational activities strengthen bonds across age groups, promoting dopamine, oxytocin, and emotional resilience. This

mirrors practices found in Blue Zones, regions with high concentrations of centenarians.

Promote Group Activities
Group endeavors—whether physical (e.g., walking groups) or mental (e.g., study groups)—boost dopamine and endorphins, enhancing motivation and happiness.

Create Spaces for Reflection and Meditation
Designated spaces for spiritual practices allow individuals to connect with themselves and others, supporting serotonin and oxytocin release.

Establish Regular Routines
Ayurveda's emphasis on regularity can be applied to community life. Consistent mealtimes, social activities, and communal events promote dosha balance and reduce stress.

Integrate Group Meditation
Implementing the Maharishi Effect through group meditation can create collective coherence, reducing stress and enhancing peace in society.

Collective Consciousness and Longevity

Social bonds, shared rituals, and collective meditation create a feedback loop that influences neurotransmitter balance, fostering health, happiness, and longevity. Collective consciousness is not just a concept but a practical path to enhancing both individual and community well-being.

As Carlos' story illustrates, reconnecting with community and engaging in collective consciousness can transform lives, fostering a sense of unity, purpose, and joy. By integrating these principles, individuals can create lasting changes within themselves and their communities, promoting both personal and collective well-being.

PART IV

APPENDICES

APPENDIX 1

ENERGY STATE CHARACTERISTICS

V (Vata) Energy State

V Energy State individuals are bright, good at creating new ideas and projects, and able to learn quickly. If, however, they become imbalanced, they may easily lose their energy and can become fatigued and oversensitive. They may also experience mood swings, and they will then have difficulty in following a project through to the end. The secret for a V person to maintain balance is to follow a good routine. Certain simple dietary and lifestyle changes will also greatly help to rebalance and sustain a V Energy State person.

The appetite of a V person tends to be irregular and their digestive power is strong at one time and weak at another. Everyone likes to snack, but a V benefits from eating several small but nutritious meals throughout the day, rather than three "solids." It is especially important for a V to eat in a quiet environment, away from distractions and stress. When their gut is balanced, the V digestion is quite good. When the V gut is out of balance, the individual may experience symptoms such as indigestion, gas, and constipation.

See *The Rest And Repair Diet: Heal Your Gut, Improve Your Physical and Mental Health, and Lose Weight* for details about specific dietary recommendations for your Energy State.

V individuals enjoy exercise that involves moving quickly and/or gracefully, but their physiology is not suited for endurance sports. They are sprinters rather than marathoners and must be very careful to not get overtired. Activities like dancing, paddleboarding, yoga—anything that keeps them moving easily—is excellent for a V. They do well with a gentle-to-moderate, grounding, warming workout.

V Energy State people frequently have a hard time going to sleep and are very susceptible to insomnia. They need to understand that they must avoid excessive stimulation before bedtime and take real steps to wind down and relax, such as having a warm bath, listening to peaceful music, and using calming aromatherapy.

P (Pitta) Energy State

P Energy State individuals tend to be well-organized and purposeful. They often possess good energy and a strong and penetrating intellect, and can be good leaders. It is no coincidence that businesspeople and athletes are frequently P individuals. When a P is imbalanced, they may have trouble controlling their anger, or, at the very least, irritation, from time to time. They can also be impatient, difficult to interact with, and controlling. The key to a P keeping in good balance is for them to eat on time and not become overheated. It's that simple!

The defining characteristic of the P Energy State is a strong digestive fire. The digestive power of all Energy States is strongest at noon, and it is best for all of them to eat their largest and heaviest meal at this time. But the P gut is programmed to produce an especially powerful appetite, so it's necessary for them to eat a good amount, on time, every day, or they will experience physical discomfort, and quite possibly, emotional turmoil or anger. When the P gut is balanced, digestion is highly efficient; but when it is out of balance, the person can experience hyperacidity and indigestion.

P Energy State individuals are usually highly competitive, and they don't hold back. Possessing stamina and strength, they are often drawn to organized sports. They are also goal-oriented and often overdo exercise, paying the consequences later. Above all, P people need to avoid becoming overheated. Active water sports like swimming, surfing, and canoeing are all good for them. If you see somebody out parasailing, that person will almost certainly prove to be a P Energy State type.

A P Energy State person tends to go to sleep quickly. But when the P person goes out of balance, he or she can experience difficulty sleeping.

K (Kapha) Energy State

K Energy State people tend to be steady and take some time to carefully consider any decision. They are not easily upset, and are often easygoing and agreeable. If they go out of balance, however, they can become stubborn and may seem to lack ambition. The key to keeping a K person in good balance is to keep them physically active and mentally stimulated.

K Energy State individuals have a good steady, digestion, and it doesn't bother them to miss an occasional meal. The K Energy

State person loves food, but because they have a slower metabolism, they will gain weight easily, and must be careful to eat only moderate amounts.

K individuals generally have good endurance and strength, and regular active physical exercise is necessary to keep them from becoming overweight and lethargic (i.e. couch potatoes). Running, jogging, and energetic gym workouts are all very beneficial.

K Energy State individuals almost never have trouble falling asleep, but they often have a hard time getting up in the morning.

VP or PV Energy State

A VP Energy State person is similar to a PV Energy State, but in written form, whichever Energy State is listed first is the one that predominates. A VP person is quick, inspiring, and full of new ideas, but at the same time is also focused and ready to complete the project. VPs can be both energetic and sensitive. One part of them is in motion, while the other is steadily goal-oriented.

When VPs are in good balance, they draw energy from their P qualities. When they are out of balance, their V qualities can cause them to become over-stimulated and quickly exhausted. This duality produces a reasonably strong but variable energy.

The digestion of a VP is like their energy, good but variable, and their appetite is similar. Because their gut is partially V, they may be a discriminating eater with strong preferences, and can be hungry one minute and not interested in food the next. But because their gut is also partially P, they need ample meals to sustain physical and mental activity. The presence of P indicates that it is especially important for VP individuals to eat on time. As a combination type, they have a more balanced appetite than people with either a pure V or a pure P Energy State.

When VPs are in good balance, they rarely have digestive problems. When out of balance, however, digestive issues can range from weak digestion to hyperacidity.

VP Energy State people are agile and have good energy and strength. They may also tend to be graceful. VP Energy individuals do not have a problem falling asleep unless they are over-stimulated before going to bed.

VK or KV Energy State

This Energy State is an interesting combination of opposites. The V Energy State is light and airy, while the K Energy State is heavy and earthy. This combination indicates both steadiness and enthusiasm.

When VK is in good balance, the result is good health and physical stamina. When it is out of balance, VK people are prone to frequent colds and respiratory problems. With this particular energy state, it's important to remember that an imbalance of V will always push K out of balance, so V imbalances need to be addressed as soon as possible. VKs don't do well in cold or damp weather and need to stay warm to avoid illness.

The VK combination gives rise to individuals who have a wide range of emotions. They are quick, inspiring, and full of new ideas, but at the same time they are stable, well liked, and methodical. VKs can be both grounded and sensitive. One part of them is in constant airy motion, while the other is steady and grounded.

When out of balance, a VK person tends to be spacey, withdrawn, or even depressed. They may also obsess on issues and become attached and/or anxious. It's especially good for VKs to have enjoyable social outings and to stay rested, as well as energized, in order to balance the best aspects of their mind, body, and emotions.

The digestion of a VK Energy State person is virtually the same as a KV Energy State person. Again, as we mentioned, the energy state listed first indicates which is predominant. VKs are generally strong and steady, and enjoy an occasional snack. The V part of the VK combination makes the person a grazer, with a constantly changing appetite, while their K part makes them love to eat. When they are in good balance, V and K complement each other very well. They enjoy food, but don't gain as much weight as pure K types until later in life.

When out of balance, the VK, KV digestion slows down and they become more sensitive to what they eat.

In regard to exercise, VK Energy State individuals are a mixture of opposites and may be sprinters as well as endurance runners.

VK Energy individuals can fall asleep and stay asleep as long as their V Energy State is balanced.

PK or KP Energy State

PK Energy State people have the hot, transformative qualities of a P Energy State plus the cool, stable qualities of a K Energy State.

If they are unable to stay in balance, however, they can boil over. PKs are generally large and strong and do well in sports. Many professional athletes are PK. They might not be the stars of the team, but they have the constitution to be very good players.

A PK tends to be strong, sturdy, content, and easygoing. Their high energy drive is steadied by their calm, easygoing nature. Imbalances can cause impatience, anger, and lethargy. They may also become argumentative, stubborn, and withdrawn. It's very important for a PK particularly to maintain healthy family relationships and friendships in order to stay in good balance.

In the heat of the moment a PK might not think problems through completely. And if decisions backfire, they may be prone to useless regret. A PK individual will be happier and healthier spending more time listening and less time making assumptions and running scenarios in their head.

The PK digestion and appetite is virtually the same as KP. In both cases, each of the combined energy states is strong, but P will predominate. People with a P gut have a good appetite, and strong digestion. If they have a PK gut, they will have an even stronger appetite. PKs like to eat, and generally digest easily. Because their gut is part K, however, their metabolism slows down at times and they may have a hard time digesting greasy foods. It's easy for PKs to gain a few extra pounds, but they can usually lose them without great effort.

When PKs are in good balance, they rarely have digestive problems. When out of balance, however, they must be aware of slower digestion and hyperacidity.

PKs need to exercise daily. They have excellent stamina in activity, but must remember not to get overheated. The PK or KP individual generally falls asleep easily and gets a good sound sleep.

VPK Energy State or "Tri-Energy State"

This is a relatively rare mixture of the three types and, when it is in balance, shows the best qualities of each. VPKs are often creative, motivated, steady, and good-natured. When they are in good balance, they tend to be in tune with their body and emotions and may be intuitive. Physically strong with a moderate build, VPKs are usually in good health. They avoid most seasonal illnesses and experience only mild to moderate symptoms during each season (e.g. dry skin in the winter, some lethargy in the spring, and mild heat intolerance in the summer).

Life for a VPK becomes complicated when one or more of their three Energy States goes out of balance and it is helpful for them to learn to "check in" with themselves and be alert to when something doesn't feel right. The best advice for VPKs is to treat any imbalances in the following order:

- Start by balancing V

- Go on to balance P

- Finally address K

Keep in mind that it takes a VPK Energy State person longer to come back into balance than the other Energy State combinations.

The digestion and appetite of a VPK Energy State person should be good since they have a stronger digestion than others. They can eat almost any kind of food and rarely experience excessive hunger or thirst. However, because their symptoms are usually mild and somewhat veiled, it is hard to pinpoint how and when they go out of balance, so it's especially valuable for them to learn to listen to their body.

Possessing all three characteristics, they are capable of different types of exercise. The main thing is to not overdo it. Because of their K Energy State, sleep is their friend. If they do go out of balance, it is usually the V Energy State which causes a sleep problem.

Energy State Conclusion

No single Energy State is better than another and each of us can rise to our full potential by staying in balance and achieving maximum levels of energy, performance, and success. For recommendations about specific Energy State diets, including teas, spice mixes, and recipes, see The Rest and Repair Diet: Heal Your Gut, Improve Your Physical and Mental Health, and Lose Weight, and visit docgut.com.

Scientific Research on Ayurveda and Energy States

Recent studies have shown that there is a scientific basis to Ayurveda and its evaluation of each person's Energy State or Prakriti. There is a whole new field emerging called Ayurgenomics. Genetic research, for example, has shown that the Vata (V Energy State), Pitta (P Energy State), and Kapha (K Energy State) Prakriti each expresses a different set of genes. See scientific references 1 and 2 in the list below.

Genes in the immune response pathways, for example, were turned on or up-regulated in extreme Pittas. In Vatas, genes related to cell cycles were turned on. In Kaphas it was found that genes in the immune signaling pathways were turned on. Inflammatory genes were up-regulated in Vatas, whereas up-regulation of oxidative stress pathway genes was observed in Pittas and Kaphas. See reference number 3 below. CD25 (activated B cells) and CD56 (natural killer cells) were higher in Kaphas. CYP2C19 genotypes, a family of genes that help in detoxification and metabolism of certain drugs, were turned off or down-regulated in Kapha types and turned on in Pitta types. See references 4 and 5 below.

Extreme Vata, Pitta, and Kapha individuals also have significant differences in specific physiological measurements. Again, see references 1 and 2 below. Triglycerides, total cholesterol, high low-density lipoprotein (LDL), and low high-density lipoprotein (HDL) concentrations—all common risk factors for cardiovascular disease—were reported to be higher in Kaphas compared to Vatas. Hemoglobin and red blood cell count were higher in Pittas compared to others. Serum prolactin was higher in Vata individuals. See reference 2 below. High levels of triglyceride, VLDL and LDL levels and lower levels of HDL cholesterol distinguish Kaphas from others. See reference 6 below.

Adenosine diphosphate-induced maximal platelet aggregation was the highest among Vata/Pitta types. See reference 7 below. In diabetic patients, there were significant decreases in systolic blood pressure in Vata/Pitta, Pitta/Kapha, and Vata/Kapha types after walking (isotonic exercise). The Vata/Pitta types also showed significant decreases in mean diastolic blood pressure. See reference 8 below. In terms of biochemistry, Kaphas had elevated digoxin levels, increased free radical production, and reduced scavenging, increased tryptophan catabolites and reduced tyrosine catabolites, increased glycoconjugate levels, and increased cholesterol. Pittas showed the opposite biochemical patterns. Vatas showed normal biochemical patterns. See reference 9 below.

A study of basic cardiovascular responses reported that heart rate variability and arterial blood pressure during specific postural changes, exercise, and cold pressor test did not vary with constitutional type. See reference 10 below. A more recent paper measuring cold pressor test, standing-to-lying ratio, and pupillary responses in light and dark reported that Kapha types have higher parasympathetic activity and lower sympathetic activity in terms of cardiovascular reactivity as compared to Pitta or Vata types. See reference 11 below.

A recent study also showed that predominantly Vata, Pitta, or Kapha people had a different composition of bacteria in their microbiome. See reference 12 and 13 below. Sharma and Wallace in an article entitled *Ayurveda and Epigenetics* (reference 14) have shown how the time-tested lifestyle recommendations of Ayurveda act as epigenetic regulators to create balance in the physiology. Finally, Travis and Wallace have reviewed many of these findings, and created a neurophysiological model of Vata, Pitta, and Kapha based on the functioning of different neural networks. See reference 15 below.

Selected References

1. Dey S, Pahwa P. Prakriti and its associations with metabolism, chronic diseases, and genotypes: Possibilities of new born screening and a lifetime of personalized prevention. J Ayurveda Integr Med 2014;5:15-24.

2. Wallace, RK. Ayurgenomics and Modern Medicine. Medicina 2020, 56, 661.

3. Juyal RC, Negi S, Wakhode P, Bhat S, Bhat B, Thelma BK. Potential of ayurgenomics approach in complex trait research: Leads from a pilot study on rheumatoid arthritis. PLoS One. 2012;7:e45752.

4. Ghodke Y, Joshi K, Patwardhan B. Traditional medicine to modern pharmacogenomics: Ayurveda Prakriti type and CYP2C19 gene polymorphism associated with the metabolic variability. Evid Based Complement Alternat Med 2011;2011:249528.

5. Aggarwal S, Negi S, Jha P, Singh PK, Stobdan T, Pasha MA. Indian genome variation consortium. EGLN1 involvement in high-altitude adaptation revealed through genetic analysis of extreme constitution types defined in Ayurveda. Proc Natl Acad Sci 2010;107:18961-6.

6. Mahalle NP, Kulkarni MV, Pendse NM, Naik SS. Association of constitutional type of Ayurveda with cardiovascular risk factors, inflammatory markers and insulin resistance. J Ayurveda Integr Med 2012;3:150-7.

7. Bhalerao S, Deshpande T, Thatte U. Prakriti (Ayurvedic concept of constitution) and variations in Platelet aggregation. BMC Complement Altern Med 2012;12:248-56.

8. Tiwari S, Gehlot S, Tiwari SK, Singh G. Effect of walking (aerobic isotonic exercise) on physiological variants with special reference to Prameha (diabetes mellitus) as per Prakriti. Ayu 2012;33:44-9.

9. Kurup RK, Kurup PA. Hypothalamic digoxin, hemispheric chemical dominance, and the tridosha theory. Int J Neurosci 2003;113:657-81.

10. Tripathi PK, Patwardhan K, Singh G. The basic cardiovascular responses to postural changes, exercise and cold pressor test: Do they vary in accordance with the dual constitutional types of Ayurveda? Evid Based Complement Alternat Med 2011;201:251-9.

11. Rapolu SB, Kumar M, Singh G, Patwardhan K. Physiological

variations in the autonomic responses may be related to the constitutional types defined in Ayurveda. J Humanitas Med 2015;5:e7.

12. Chauhan NS, Pandey R, Mondal AK, Gupta S, Verma MK, Jain S, et al. Western Indian Rural Gut Microbial Diversity in Extreme Prakriti Endo-Phenotypes Reveals Signature Microbes. Front. Microbiol. 2018; 9:118. doi: 10.3389/fmicb.2018.00118. eCollection 2018.

13. Wallace, RK. The Microbiome in Health and Disease from the Perspective of Modern Medicine and Ayurveda. Medicina 2020; 56, 462.

14. Sharma, H.; Wallace, RK. Ayurveda and Epigenetics. Medicina 2020; 56, 687.

15. Travis, FT, Wallace. RK, Dosha brain-types: A neural model of individual differences. J Ayurveda Integr Med. 2015; 6, 280-85.

APPENDIX 2

AYURVEDIC DIET AND DIGESTION

General Ayurvedic Principles for Eating

In addition to dosha-specific dietary recommendations, Ayurveda emphasizes several key principles for maintaining optimal digestion and health:

- Eat your largest meal at midday:

- Digestion is strongest when the sun is at its peak, making lunch the best time to consume heavier meals.

- Sit while eating: Eating in a calm, settled environment improves digestion and allows the body to properly process food.

- Avoid overeating: Ayurveda recommends eating until you are about three-quarters full, allowing room for digestion to occur smoothly.

- Sip warm water during meals: Cold drinks, especially ice water, extinguish the digestive fire (Agni). Warm water aids digestion and supports nutrient absorption.

- Avoid snacking between meals: Allowing time between meals helps digestion complete its process, preventing the accumulation of Ama.

- Choose fresh, organic foods: Fresh, organic produce and whole foods are considered more nourishing and free of harmful toxins. Ayurveda also encourages consuming foods that are locally grown and in season.

General Dietary Recommendations for Vata, Pitta, and Kapha

Ayurveda offers specific dietary guidelines to balance each dosha. The idea is to consume foods that counterbalance the inherent qualities of each dosha to maintain harmony within the body and mind.

Vata Diet (Balancing Air and Space):
Vata types often have sensitive digestion, with a tendency toward constipation, gas, and bloating. They benefit from warm, grounding, and moist foods that stabilize their airy, mobile nature.

Foods to favor:
Warm, cooked foods like soups, stews, cooked grains, and roasted nuts. Sweet, sour, and salty tastes are recommended to pacify Vata. Fats like ghee, olive oil, and nuts are also balancing.

Foods to avoid:
Cold, raw, dry, and light foods such as salads, crackers, and raw vegetables. These foods can aggravate Vata's dryness and lead to digestive imbalances.

Neurotransmitter focus:
Vata types should focus on foods that support dopamine production to enhance focus and reduce scattered energy. Warm,

cooked meals that include healthy fats are particularly beneficial for Vata's nervous system.

Pitta Diet (Balancing Fire and Water):

Pitta types have strong digestion but are prone to overheating and inflammation. They benefit from cooling, soothing foods that calm their fiery nature and prevent digestive and emotional burnouts.

Foods to favor:

Cooling, sweet, and bitter foods like cucumbers, leafy greens, coconut water, and dairy products (if tolerated). Rice, oats, and wheat are also beneficial.

Foods to avoid:

Spicy, sour, salty, and oily foods, which can increase Pitta's heat and lead to issues like heartburn, irritability, and inflammation. Excessive caffeine and alcohol should also be minimized.

Neurotransmitter focus:

Pitta types should prioritize foods that balance serotonin and GABA to maintain emotional calm and prevent stress-related issues.

Kapha Diet (Balancing Earth and Water):

Kapha types tend to have slower digestion and metabolism, which can lead to weight gain and lethargy. They benefit from light, stimulating foods that energize and increase metabolism.

Foods to favor:

Light, dry, and spicy foods like ginger, lentils, and leafy greens. Pungent and astringent tastes, such as those found in bitter greens and spices, are balancing for Kapha.

Foods to avoid:

Heavy, oily, and sweet foods like dairy, fried foods, and sugary snacks, which can slow down digestion and exacerbate Kapha imbalances.

Neurotransmitter focus:

Kapha types should focus on foods that stimulate dopamine production to increase motivation and reduce emotional sluggishness. Spices and lighter meals are key to keeping Kapha balanced and energized.

Specific Recommendations for Vata, Pitta, and Kapha

Vata Diet

- Sip hot water throughout the day to promote natural detoxing and improve digestion.

- An ideal breakfast is cooked cereal with roasted nuts and a little fruit. If you're gluten intolerant, pick appropriate non-gluten grains.

- Roasted nuts and seeds are good, especially almonds. It's best not to eat raw nuts, but we can only do what we can do. Roasting nuts helps with digestion and assimilation. Ayurveda recommends first soaking them overnight and then roasting.

- All fresh organic dairy products are highly recommended.

- A modest amount of any natural sweetener helps to calm Vata.

- Hot cooked food is better for a Vata than cold or uncooked food.

- Small leafy salads, however, are OK.

- Favor rice and, if you can, wheat, and oats (cooked, not dry).

- Eating fresh corn in season is fine! Otherwise, not so much.

- Reduce your intake of millet, barley, buckwheat, and rye.

- A Vata is vulnerable to excess gas, so reduce the intake of all bean products accordingly. (Tofu is hard to digest. But if you love it, then take small amounts, and only if it's very fresh.)

- Fruits should be very ripe, sweet, and juicy!

- For non-vegetarians, favor fresh organic chicken, turkey, fish, and eggs.

- Avoid stimulants like coffee, tea, and other caffeine-laden beverages. Try to cool it on the alcohol.

If you've been using skim milk to reduce your fat intake, ayurvedic doctors recommend that you buy organic whole milk and dilute it with purified water. This will reduce your fat intake but will also ensure that you benefit from the important synergistic value of all the nutrients in the milk.

If you're not sleeping well, cook a cup of whole milk for several minutes (ideally, bring it to a boil four times). While the milk is cooking, add cardamom, cinnamon, nutmeg, and coconut sugar, to taste. Drink while it's still nicely warm, but not too hot. If you find that the milk clogs you up overnight, then add a little powdered ginger to the mix. (Too much ginger can be over-stimulating and keep you up or give you a stomachache.)

Best veggies:

Best veggies include asparagus, beets, cucumbers, green beans, okra, radishes, sweet potatoes, turnips, carrots, and artichokes. Other vegetables may be eaten in moderation if cooked in ghee (clarified butter) or extra-virgin olive oil. Avoid or reduce cabbage, cauliflower, Brussels sprouts, or bean sprouts. No raw vegetables except for small leafy salads.

Best fruits:

Best fruits include apricots, plums, berries, melons, papayas, peaches, cherries, nectarines, and bananas. Also good are dates, figs, pineapples, and mangoes. If you have digestive problems, fruits are best eaten lightly stewed or sautéed. Avocados (technically a fruit) are very good for Vatas.

Best spices:

Best spices include basil, cardamom, cilantro, cinnamon, clove, cumin, fennel, fenugreek, ginger, licorice root, marjoram, nutmeg, oregano, sage, tarragon, and thyme. Allspice, anise, asafoetida, bay leaf, caraway, juniper berries, mace, and mustard can be used with discretion. Use black pepper sparingly. Minimize or eliminate all bitter and astringent spices.

Pitta Diet

- Organic grains like wheat, rice, barley, and oats are good. Reduce your consumption of corn, rye, millet, and brown rice.

- Most nuts are not good for a Pitta. Pumpkin seeds and sunflower seeds are alright.

- Favor organic coconut, olive, and sunflower oils.

- Avoid almond, corn, safflower, and sesame oils.

- Favor mung beans and chickpeas.

- Tofu and other soy products should be fresh. (In Japan, it's not uncommon for people to refuse tofu products that are more than a day old.)

- For non-vegetarians, organic free-range chicken and turkey are preferable to red meat and seafood.

Best veggies:

Best veggies include asparagus, potatoes, sweet potatoes, leafy greens, broccoli, cauliflower, celery, okra, lettuce, green beans, peas, and zucchini. Also good are Brussels sprouts, cabbage, cucumbers, mushrooms, sprouts, and sweet peppers. Avoid or reduce tomatoes, hot peppers, onions, garlic, and hot radishes.

Best fruits:

Best fruits include apples, grapes, melons, cherries, coconuts, avocados, mangoes, pineapples, figs, oranges, and plums are recommended. Also good are prunes, and raisins. Reduce or eliminate sour fruits such as grapefruit, cranberries, lemons, and persimmons.

Best spices:

Best spices include coriander, cilantro, cardamom, and saffron. Turmeric, dill, fennel, and mint are also fine. Spices such as ginger, black pepper, fenugreek, clove, salt, and mustard seed may be used sparingly. Completely avoid pungent hot spices such as chili peppers and cayenne.

Kapha Diet

- Honey is the only sweetener that helps a Kapha. Avoid all others.

- According to Ayurveda, honey should not be heated.

- Favor barley, corn, millet, buckwheat, and rye.

- Reduce your intake of oats, rice, and wheat.

- Beans of all kinds are good for a Kapha, except kidney beans and soybeans. Soy is quite difficult to digest, and the older it is, the harder it is to digest.

- Except for pumpkin seeds and sunflower seeds, reduce or eliminate the intake of nuts and seeds.

- Use small amounts of extra virgin olive oil, ghee, almond oil, sunflower oil, or safflower oil. Steam or roast, if possible.

- Non-vegetarians should favor fresh organic free-range chicken and turkey.

Best veggies:

Best veggies include asparagus, beets, broccoli, Brussels sprouts, cabbage, carrots, cauliflower, celery, eggplant, leafy greens, lettuce, mushrooms, okra, onions, peas, peppers, potatoes, spinach, sprouts Use small amounts of ghee or extra-virgin olive oil. Reduce/Avoid: sweet potatoes, tomatoes, cucumbers, zucchini.

Best fruits:

Best fruits include pomegranates, apples, apricots, cranberries, pears. Reduce/Avoid: avocados, bananas, oranges, peaches, coconuts, melons, dates, figs, grapefruits, grapes, mangoes, papayas, plums, pineapples.

Best spices:

Best spices include ginger, horseradish, mustard, cardamom, garlic, cloves, turmeric, cayenne and peppers of all kinds. Ginger is great for improving digestion! Reduce or avoid salt.

Diet as the Key to Balance and Longevity

In Ayurveda, diet is the cornerstone of health, longevity, and emotional well-being. By following a diet that supports your dosha and aligns with your individual needs, you can optimize digestion, balance neurotransmitters, and enhance mental clarity.

The Ayurvedic approach to food is deeply personal and rooted in an understanding of the body's natural rhythms. When we eat in harmony with our unique constitution, we can unlock the full potential of our mind and body, ensuring long-lasting health and vitality.

Selected References

1. Living in Balance with Maharishi AyurVeda: Practical Therapies for Consciousness-Based Health by Robert Keith Wallace, PhD, Karin Pirc, MD, Julia Clarke, MS, MIU Press, 2023

2. The Rest And Repair Diet: Heal Your Gut, Improve Your Physical and Mental Health, and Lose Weight by Robert Keith Wallace, PhD, Samantha Wallace, Andrew Sternberg, MA Jim Davis, DO, and Alexis Farley, Dharma Publications, 2019

APPENDIX 3

TRANSCENDENTAL MEDITATION

The Transcendental Meditation technique is a unique, simple, and effective mental procedure. It takes about twenty minutes, twice each day, sitting comfortably with your eyes closed. It involves no belief or philosophy, no mood or lifestyle. Most people begin the technique for practical reasons, such as a desire for more energy or to decrease tension and anxiety. Over ten million people of all ages, cultures, and religions have learned TM.

TM uses the natural tendency of the mind to spontaneously experience states of greater and greater happiness. The technique involves a real and measurable process of physiological refinement that utilizes the inherent capacity of the nervous system to refine its own functioning and unfold its full potential. During TM practice, your attention is very naturally and spontaneously drawn to quieter, more orderly states of mental activity until all mental activity is transcended, and you are left with no thoughts or sensations, only the experience of pure awareness itself. The result of the regular practice of TM is that your entire nervous system becomes rejuvenated and revitalized, and you become more successful and fulfilled in activity.

Extensive research documents the effectiveness of TM in improving both physical and mental health. TM produces a unique state of restful alertness (2-4) with brain wave patterns that are different from other techniques of meditation (1). The practice of this technique helps every area of life by removing stress from the nervous system. Over 600 studies at more than 200 research institutes and universities have been conducted on the Transcendental Meditation program, and more than 380 of these studies have been published in peer-reviewed journals. [Note to Reader: "Peer-reviewed" means that scientists, whose qualifications and competencies are on a similar level of accomplishment as those of the authors of the study, have evaluated the work. This method is the gold standard of science, employed to maintain the highest standard of quality and credibility.]

The US National Institutes of Health has awarded over $25 million to study the effects of TM on health, particularly on heart disease, the #1 killer in the US. It is particularly interesting to note that researchers who conducted an important study at the Medical College of Wisconsin in Milwaukee reported that the more regularly the patients meditated, the longer was their term of survival (5).

A number of important studies have shown that TM reduces high blood pressure (6). A statement from the American Heart Association concluded:

> The Transcendental Meditation technique is the only meditation practice that has been shown to lower blood pressure.
>
> Because of many negative studies or mixed results and a paucity of available trials, all other meditation techniques (including MBSR) received a 'Class III, no benefit, Level of Evidence C' recommendation. Thus, other meditation techniques are not recommended in clinical practice to lower BP at this time.

> Transcendental Meditation practice is recom-
> mended for consideration in treatment plans for all
> individuals with blood pressure > 120/80 mm Hg.

> Lower blood pressure through Transcendental
> Meditation practice is also associated with sub-
> stantially reduced rates of death, heart attack,
> and stroke (7).

Research shows that TM practice reduces cholesterol levels (8). Studies also show that meditators exhibit an improved ability to adapt to stressful situations (9,10) and a marked decrease in levels of plasma cortisol, commonly known as the "stress hormone" (11).

Research results in various areas of health document improvements in such conditions as asthma, diabetes, metabolic syndrome, pain, alcohol and drug abuse, and mental health (12-17). In a five-year study on some 2000 individuals, researchers showed that TM meditators used medical and surgical health care services approximately one-half as often as did other insurance users. This study was conducted in cooperation with Blue Cross Blue Shield and controlled for other factors that might affect health care use, such as cost sharing, age, gender, geographic distribution, and profession. The TM subjects also showed a far lower rate of increase in health care utilization with increasing age (18).

In Québec, Canada, researchers compared the changes in physician costs for TM practitioners with those of non-practitioners over a five-year period. This study is particularly reliable because the Canadian government tracked health care costs closely for both meditators and the control group, due to Canada's national health care system. After the first year, the health care costs of the TM group decreased 11%, and after five years, their cumulative cost reduction was 28%. TM patients required fewer referrals, resulting in lower medical expenses for prescription drugs, tests, hospitalization, surgery, and other treatments (19).

Studies have documented how TM can slow and even reverse the aging process. One study showed that long-term TM meditators had a biological age roughly twelve years younger than their non-meditating counterparts (20). Researchers at Harvard University studied the effects of TM on mental health, behavioral flexibility, blood pressure, and longevity, in residents of homes for the elderly. The subjects were randomly assigned either to a no-treatment group or to one of three treatment programs: the TM program, mindfulness training, or a relaxation program. Initially, all three groups were similar on pretest measures and expectancy of benefits, yet after only three months, the TM group showed significant improvements in cognitive functioning and blood pressure compared to the control groups. Reports from the TM subjects, compared to those of the mindfulness or the relaxation subjects, indicated that the TM practitioners felt more absorbed during their practice, and better and more relaxed immediately afterward. Overall, more TM subjects found their practice to be personally valuable than members of either of the control groups (21).

The most striking finding is that TM practice not only reverses age-related declines in overall health, but also directly enhances longevity. All the members of the TM group were still alive three years after the program began, in contrast to about only half of the members of the control groups. Research on the Transcendental Meditation program clearly shows that growing old can be an opportunity for further development (22,23). Scientists have suggested that one of the ways TM may improve health and increase longevity is by changing the expression of specific beneficial genes in our DNA (24,25).

Long-term changes in brain functioning have also been correlated with decreased stress-reactivity and neuroticism, and increased self-development, intelligence, learning ability, and self-actualization (26-30). One important psychological study on TM shows a significant decrease in levels of anxiety in TM practitioners as compared to subjects practicing other relaxation techniques (31). Studies in a variety of work and business settings show significantly increased productivity and efficiency (32,33). A recent study showed marked improvements in veterans with PTSD (34).

TM is learned from a qualified TM teacher, and is taught in 7 steps, usually within a week's time according to your schedule. Most of the steps take 1 to 2 hours (though some are shorter). There is also a brief but important follow-up meeting 10 days after you learn the practice, and then once a month for the first three months after your TM course. All of these meetings are included in the course fee, along with lifelong support for your meditation program, including individual meditation checking, advanced meetings, and other special events.

Although there are a number of advanced TM programs, TM is always the core technique and will continue to benefit your life whether you choose to take an advanced program or not. (For more information on how to start TM, see TM.org.)

Selected References

1. Travis FT and Shear J. Focused attention, open monitoring and automatic self-transcending: Categories to organize meditations from

Vedic, Buddhist and Chinese traditions. Consciousness and Cognition 19(4):1110-1118, 2010

2. Wallace RK. Physiological effects of Transcendental Meditation. Science 167:1751-1754, 1970

3. Wallace RK, et al. A wakeful hypometabolic physiologic state. American Journal of Physiology 221(3): 795-799, 1971

4. Wallace RK. Physiological effects of the Transcendental Meditation technique: A proposed fourth major state of consciousness. Ph.D. thesis. Physiology Department, University of California, Los Angeles, 1970

5. Schneider RH, et al. Stress Reduction in the Secondary Prevention of Cardiovascular Disease: Randomized, Controlled Trial of Transcendental Meditation and Health Education in Blacks. Circ Cardiovasc Qual Outcomes 5:750-758, 2012

6. Rainforth MV, et al. Stress reduction programs in patients with elevated blood pressure: a systematic review and meta-analysis. Current Hypertension Reports 9:520–528, 2007

7. Brook RD, et al., Beyond Medications and Diet: Alternative Approaches to Lowering Blood Pressure. A Scientific Statement from the American Heart Association. Hypertension 61(6):1360-83, 2013

8. Cooper MJ, et al. Transcendental Meditation in the management of hypercholesterolemia. Journal of Human Stress 5(4): 24–27, 1979

9. Orme-Johnson DW and Walton KW. All approaches of preventing or reversing effects of stress are not the same. American Journal of Health Promotion 12:297-299, 1998

10. Barnes VA, et al. Impact of Transcendental Meditation on cardiovascular function at rest and during acute stress in adolescents with high normal blood pressure. Journal of Psychosomatic Research 51: 597-605, 2001

11. Jevning R, et al. Adrenocortical activity during meditation. Hormonal Behavior 10(1):54-60, 1978

12. Wilson AF, et al. Transcendental Meditation and asthma. Respiration 32:74-80, 1975

13. Paul-Labrador M, et al. Effects of randomized controlled trial of Transcendental Meditation on components of the metabolic syndrome

in subjects with coronary heart disease. Archives of Internal Medicine 166:1218-1224, 2006

14. Royer A. The role of the Transcendental Meditation technique in promoting smoking cessation: A longitudinal study. Alcoholism Treatment Quarterly 11: 219-236, 1994

15. Haratani T, et al. Effects of Transcendental Meditation (TM) on the mental health of industrial workers. Japanese Journal of Industrial Health 32: 656, 1990

16. Orme-Johnson DW, et al. Neuroimaging of meditation's effect on brain reactivity to pain. NeuroReport 17(12):1359-63, 2006

17. Alexander CN, et al. Treating and preventing alcohol, nicotine, and drug abuse through Transcendental Meditation: A review and statistical meta-analysis. Alcoholism Treatment Quarterly 11: 13-87, 1994

18. Orme-Johnson DW, Herron RE. An Innovative Approach to Reducing Medical Care Utilization and Expenditures. American Journal of Managed Care 3: 135–144, 1997

19. Herron RE. Can the Transcendental Meditation Program Reduce the Medical Expenditures of Older People? A Longitudinal Cost-Reduction Study in Canada. Journal of Social Behavior and Personality 17(1): 415–442, 2005

20. Wallace RK, et al. The effects of the Transcendental Meditation and TM-Sidhi program on the aging process. International Journal of Neuroscience 16: 53-58, 1982

21. Alexander CN, et al. Transcendental Meditation, mindfulness, and longevity. Journal of Personality and Social Psychology 57: 950-964, 1989

22. Alexander CN, et al. The effects of Transcendental Meditation compared to other methods of relaxation in reducing risk factors, morbidity, and mortality. Homeostasis 35: 243-264, 1994

23. Schneider RH, et al. Long-term effects of stress reduction on mortality in persons > 55 years of age with systemic hypertension. American Journal of Cardiology 95: 1060-1064, 2005

24. Duraimani S, et al. Effects of Lifestyle Modification on Telomerase Gene Expression in Hypertensive Patients: A Pilot Trial of Stress Reduction and Health Education Programs in African Americans. PLOS

ONE 10(11): e0142689, 2015

25. Wenuganen S, Walton KG, Katta S, Dalgard CL, Sukumar G, Starr J, Travis FT, Wallace RK, Morehead P, Lonsdorf NK, Srivastava M, Fagan J. Transcriptomics of Long-Term Meditation Practice: Evidence for Prevention or Reversal of Stress Effects Harmful to Health. Medicina (Kaunas) 57(3): 218, 2021

26. Chandler HM, et al. Transcendental Meditation and postconventional self-development: A 10-year longitudinal study. Journal of Social Behavior and Personality 17(1): 93–121, 2005

27. Cranson RW, et al. Transcendental Meditation and improved performance on intelligence-related measures: A longitudinal study. Personality and Individual Differences 12: 1105-1116, 1991

28. So KT, and Orme-Johnson DW. Three randomized experiments on the longitudinal effects of the Transcendental Meditation technique on cognition. Intelligence 29: 419-440, 2001

29. Tjoa A. Increased intelligence and reduced neuroticism through the Transcendental Meditation program. Gedrag: Tijdschrift voor Psychologie 3: 167-182, 1975

30. Alexander CN, et al. Transcendental Meditation, self-actualization, and psychological health: A conceptual overview and statistical meta-analysis. Journal of Social Behavior and Personality 6: 189-247, 1991

31. Eppley KR, et al. Differential effects of relaxation techniques on trait anxiety: A meta-analysis. Journal of Clinical Psychology 45: 957-974, 1989

32. Alexander CN, et al. Effects of the Transcendental Meditation program on stress-reduction, health, and employee development: A prospective study in two occupational settings. Stress, Anxiety and Coping 6: 245–262, 1993

33. Harung HS, et al. Peak performance and higher states of consciousness: A study of world-class performers. Journal of Managerial Psychology 11(4): 3–23, 1996

34. Nidich S, et al. Non-trauma-focused meditation versus exposure therapy in veterans with post-traumatic stress disorder: a randomised controlled trial. Lancet Psychiatry 5(12):975-986, 2018

APPENDIX 4

GROUP DYNAMICS OF CONSCIOUSNESS

Maharishi Mahesh Yogi, founder of the Transcendental Meditation technique, was the first to encourage scientific research on the concept of collective consciousness. Many scientific papers, published in peer-reviewed journals, verify the practical application of Maharishi's concepts. Many of the comments about the group dynamics of consciousness can be found in Maharishi's books.

In 1960, Maharishi predicted that one percent of a population practicing the Transcendental Meditation technique would produce measurable improvements in the quality of life for the whole population. This phenomenon was first studied in 1974 and was referred to as the "Maharishi Effect." In 1976, Maharishi brought out several advanced programs derived from the Vedic tradition, which greatly enhanced the Maharishi Effect. Scientists found that when even the square root of one percent of any population practices these programs in a group, there is a measurable marked reduction in violence and an improvement in the quality of life, a type of macroscopic field effect of coherence.

A large number of studies have documented the beneficial effects of the practice of TM and its advanced programs on reducing crime and violence and improving the quality of life in different areas of the world. One demonstration project was conducted in 1993 in Washington, DC by Dr. John Hagelin and colleagues. An independent panel of more than twenty sociologists, criminologists, and members of the Washington, DC government and police department advised on the study design and reviewed the analysis of the findings. The study included over 4000 people gathered in Washington to participate in a "peace assembly," practicing TM and specific related advanced programs for extended periods. Results showed that as the group size increased, there was a highly significant decrease in violent crime.

A remarkable aspect of this study was that it took place in the summer, when the weather is especially hot in Washington. In fact, the police chief of Washington, who sat on the independent board of researchers monitoring the project, said in an interview, "The only way this group can lower crime by 20 percent in Washington in August is if we have two feet of snow!" In fact, the meditating group lowered crime by 23.6 percent.

How could such a thing happen? The individuals in the group didn't go out on the streets and physically stop people from committing crimes. They simply meditated quietly together in various locations around the city. The coherence effect which they created in the collective consciousness of the city was similar to the result of throwing a pebble in a pond: ripples of higher, more coherent waves of consciousness went out in all directions, creating sufficient coherence in the collective consciousness of the city so that crime was spontaneously reduced.

Research demonstrates that it is possible to influence the collective consciousness of society through the group practice of the TM technique and its advanced programs.

Selected References

1. Hagelin JS, et al. Effects of group practice of the Transcendental Meditation program on preventing violent crime in Washington, DC: results of the National Demonstration Project, June-July 1993. *Social Indicators Research* 47: 153-201, 1999

2. Orme-Johnson DW, et al. International peace project in the Middle East: The effect of the Maharishi Technology of the Unified Field. *Journal of Conflict Resolution* 32: 776–812, 1988

3. Orme-Johnson DW, et al. The long-term effects of the Maharishi Technology of the Unified Field on the quality of life in the United States (1960 to 1983). *Social Science Perspectives Journal* 2:127-146, 1988

4. Orme-Johnson DW, et al. Preventing terrorism and international conflict: Effects of large assemblies of participants in the Transcendental Meditation and TM-Sidhi programs. *Journal of Offender Rehabilitation* 36: 283–302, 2003

5. Brown CL. Overcoming barriers to use of promising research among elite Middle East policy groups. *Journal of Social Behavior and Personality* 17:489-546, 2005

6. Cavanaugh KL. Time series analysis of U.S. and Canadian inflation and unemployment: A test of a field-theoretic hypothesis. *Proceedings of the American Statistical Association, Business and Economics Statistics Section* (Alexandria, VA: American Statistical Association): 799–804, 1987

7. Cavanaugh KL, King KD. Simultaneous transfer function analysis of Okun's misery index: Improvements in the economic quality of life through Maharishi's Vedic Science and technology of

consciousness. *Proceedings of the American Statistical Association, Business and Economics Statistics Section* (Alexandria, VA: American Statistical Association): 491–496, 1988

8. Davies JL. Alleviating political violence through enhancing coherence in collective consciousness. *Dissertation Abstracts International* 49(8): 2381A, 1989

9. Gelderloos P, et al. The dynamics of US–Soviet relations, 1979–1986: Effects of reducing social stress through the Transcendental Meditation and TM-Sidhi program. *Proceedings of the Social Statistics Section of the American Statistical Association* (Alexandria, VA: American Statistical Association): 297–302, 1990

10. Dillbeck MC. Test of a field theory of consciousness and social change: Time series analysis of participation in the TM-Sidhi program and reduction of violent death in the U.S. *Social Indicators Research* 22: 399–418, 1990

11. Assimakis PD, Dillbeck MC. Time series analysis of improved quality of life in Canada: Social change, collective consciousness, and the TM-Sidhi program. *Psychological Reports* 76: 1171–1193, 1995

12. Hatchard GD, et al. A model for social improvement. Time series analysis of a phase transition to reduced crime in Merseyside metropolitan area. *Psychology, Crime, and Law* 2: 165–174, 1996

13. Dillbeck MC, et al. The Transcendental Meditation program and crime rate change in a sample of forty-eight cities. *Journal of Crime and Justice* 4: 25–45, 1981

14. Dillbeck MC, et al. Test of a field model of consciousness and social change: The Transcendental Meditation and TM-Sidhi program and decreased urban crime. *The Journal of Mind and Behavior* 9: 457–486, 1988

15. Dillbeck MC. et al. Consciousness as a field: The Transcendental Meditation and TM-Sidhi program and changes in social indicators. *The Journal of Mind and Behavior* 8: 67–104, 1987.

REFERENCES

Useful Websites

totalbraincoaching.com
ayurvedapartner.com
TM.org
MIU.edu

Useful References

Introduction

Jackson M. Evaluating the Role of Hans Selye in the Modern History of Stress. In: Cantor D, Ramsden E, editors. Stress, Shock, and Adaptation in the Twentieth Century. Rochester (NY): University of Rochester Press; 2014 Feb. Chapter 1. Available from: https://www.ncbi.nlm.nih.gov/books/NBK349158/

Baik JH. Stress and the dopaminergic reward system. Exp Mol Med. 2020 Dec;52(12):1879-1890. doi: 10.1038/s12276-020-00532-4. Epub 2020 Dec 1. PMID: 33257725; PMCID: PMC8080624.

Bloomfield MA, McCutcheon RA, Kempton M, Freeman TP, Howes O. The effects of psychosocial stress on dopaminergic function and the acute stress response. Elife. 2019 Nov 12;8:e46797. doi: 10.7554/eLife.46797. PMID: 31711569; PMCID: PMC6850765. Wallace RK. Physiological effects of Transcendental Meditation. Science 167:1751-1754, 1970

Aliev G, Beeraka NM, Nikolenko VN, Svistunov AA, Rozhnova T, Kostyuk S, Cherkesov I, Gavryushova LV, Chekhonatsky AA, Mikhaleva LM, Somasundaram SG, Avila-Rodriguez MF, Kirkland CE.

Neurophysiology and Psychopathology Underlying PTSD and Recent Insights into the PTSD Therapies-A Comprehensive Review. J Clin Med. 2020 Sep 12;9(9):2951. doi: 10.3390/jcm9092951. PMID: 32932645; PMCID: PMC7565106.

Mizoguchi, K., Yuzuihara, M., Ishige, A., Sasaki, H., Chui, D.-H., Tabira, T., 2000. Chronic stress induces impairment of spatial working memory due to prefrontal dopaminergic dysfunction. J. Neurosci. 20, 1568e1575

Wallace RK. Physiological effects of the Transcendental Meditation technique: A proposed fourth major state of consciousness. Ph.D. thesis. Physiology Department, University of California, Los Angeles, 1970

Wallace, R.K.; Wallace, T. Neuroadaptability and Habit: Modern Medicine and Ayurveda. Medicina 2021, 57, 90. doi: 10.3390/medicina57020090

Chapter 1

Speranza L, di Porzio U, Viggiano D, de Donato A, Volpicelli F. Dopamine: The Neuromodulator of Long-Term Synaptic Plasticity, Reward and Movement Control. Cells. 2021 Mar 26;10(4):735. doi: 10.3390/cells10040735. PMID: 33810328; PMCID: PMC8066851.

Berke JD. What does dopamine mean? Nat Neurosci. 2018 Jun;21(6):787-793. doi: 10.1038/s41593-018-0152-y. Epub 2018 May 14. PMID: 29760524; PMCID: PMC6358212.

Chapter 2

The Molecule of More: How a Single Chemical in Your Brain Drives Love, Sex, and Creativity - And Will Determine the Fate of the Human Race by Daniel Z. Lieberman MD, Michael E. Long, ⊠ BenBella Books 2019

Teleanu RI, Niculescu AG, Roza E, Vladâcenco O, Grumezescu AM, Teleanu DM. Neurotransmitters-Key Factors in Neurological and Neurodegenerative Disorders of the Central Nervous System. Int J Mol Sci.

2022 May 25;23(11):5954. doi: 10.3390/ijms23115954. PMID: 35682631; PMCID: PMC9180936.

Chapter 3

Mapping the Mind by Rita Carter, University of California Press, 1998

The Human Brain Book: An Illustrated Guide to its Structure, Function, and Disorders by Rita Carter, DK, 2019

Beaty RE. The Creative Brain. Cerebrum. 2020 Jan 1;2020:cer-02-20. PMID: 32206175; PMCID: PMC7075500.

Chapter 4

The Molecule of More: How a Single Chemical in Your Brain Drives Love, Sex, and Creativity - And Will Determine the Fate of the Human Race

by Daniel Z. Lieberman MD, Michael E. Long, BenBella Books 2019

Chapter 5

The Molecule of More: How a Single Chemical in Your Brain Drives Love, Sex, and Creativity - And Will Determine the Fate of the Human Race

by Daniel Z. Lieberman MD, Michael E. Long, BenBella Books 2019

Chapter 6

The Molecule of More: How a Single Chemical in Your Brain Drives Love, Sex, and Creativity - And Will Determine the Fate of the Human Race

by Daniel Z. Lieberman MD, Michael E. Long, BenBella Books 2019

Chapter 7

Volkow ND, Michaelides M, Baler R. The Neuroscience of Drug Reward and Addiction. Physiol Rev. 2019 Oct 1;99(4):2115-2140. doi: 10.1152/physrev.00014.2018. PMID: 31507244; PMCID: PMC6890985.

Liu JF, Li JX. Drug addiction: a curable mental disorder? Acta Pharmacol Sin. 2018 Dec;39(12):1823-1829. doi: 10.1038/s41401-018-0180-x. Epub 2018 Oct 31. PMID: 30382181; PMCID: PMC6289334.

Alexander CN, et al. Treating and preventing alcohol, nicotine, and drug abuse through Transcendental Meditation: A review and statistical meta-analysis. Alcoholism Treatment Quarterly 11: 13-87, 1994

Chapter 8

Elton A, Faulkner ML, Robinson DL, Boettiger CA. Acute depletion of dopamine precursors in the human brain: effects on functional connectivity and alcohol attentional bias. Neuropsychopharmacology. 2021 Jul;46(8):1421-1431. doi: 10.1038/s41386-021-00993-9. Epub 2021 Mar 16. PMID: 33727642; PMCID: PMC8209208.

Chapter 9

Living in Balance with Maharishi AyurVeda: Practical Therapies for Consciousness-Based Health by Robert Keith Wallace, PhD, Karin Pirc, MD, Julia Clarke, MS, MIU Press, 2023

Sheshagiri, Srihari. Dopamine and Vata Dosha. Journal of Indian System of Medicine 11(1):p 1-7, Jan–Mar 2023. | DOI: 10.4103/jism.jism_14_23

Chapter 10

Living in Balance with Maharishi AyurVeda: Practical Therapies for

Consciousness-Based Health by Robert Keith Wallace, PhD, Karin Pirc, MD, Julia Clarke, MS, MIU Press, 2023

The Molecule of More: How a Single Chemical in Your Brain Drives Love, Sex, and Creativity - And Will Determine the Fate of the Human Race by Daniel Z. Lieberman MD, Michael E. Long, BenBella Books 2019

Ballard IC, Murty VP, Carter RM, MacInnes JJ, Huettel SA, Adcock RA. Dorsolateral prefrontal cortex drives mesolimbic dopaminergic regions to initiate motivated behavior. J Neurosci. 2011 Jul 13;31(28):10340-6. doi: 10.1523/JNEUROSCI.0895-11.2011. PMID: 21753011; PMCID: PMC3182466.

Sheshagiri, Srihari. Dopamine and Vata Dosha. Journal of Indian System of Medicine 11(1):p 1-7, Jan–Mar 2023. | DOI: 10.4103/jism.jism_14_23

Chapter 11

Living in Balance with Maharishi AyurVeda: Practical Therapies for Consciousness-Based Health by Robert Keith Wallace, PhD, Karin Pirc, MD, Julia Clarke, MS, MIU Press, 2023

The Molecule of More: How a Single Chemical in Your Brain Drives Love, Sex, and Creativity - And Will Determine the Fate of the Human Race by Daniel Z. Lieberman MD, Michael E. Long, BenBella Books 2019

Blair RJR. Considering anger from a cognitive neuroscience perspective. Wiley Interdiscip Rev Cogn Sci. 2012 Jan;3(1):65-74. doi: 10.1002/wcs.154. Epub 2011 Oct 19. PMID: 22267973; PMCID: PMC3260787.

Chapter 12

Living in Balance with Maharishi AyurVeda: Practical Therapies for Consciousness-Based Health by Robert Keith Wallace, PhD, Karin Pirc, MD, Julia Clarke, MS, MIU Press, 2023

The Molecule of More: How a Single Chemical in Your Brain Drives Love, Sex, and Creativity - And Will Determine the Fate of the Human Race by Daniel Z. Lieberman MD, Michael E. Long, BenBella Books 2019

Chapter 13

Allada R, Bass J. Circadian Mechanisms in Medicine. N Engl J Med. 2021 Feb 11;384(6):550-561. doi: 10.1056/NEJMra1802337. PMID: 33567194; PMCID: PMC8108270.

Cornelissen G, Otsuka K. Chronobiology of Aging: A Mini-Review. Gerontology. 2017;63(2):118-128. doi: 10.1159/000450945. Epub 2016 Oct 22. PMID: 27771728.

Lewis RG, Florio E, Punzo D, Borrelli E. The Brain's Reward System in Health and Disease. Adv Exp Med Biol. 2021;1344:57-69. doi: 10.1007/978-3-030-81147-1_4. PMID: 34773226; PMCID: PMC8992377.

Chapter 14

Living in Balance with Maharishi AyurVeda: Practical Therapies for Consciousness-Based Health by Robert Keith Wallace, PhD, Karin Pirc, MD, Julia Clarke, MS, MIU Press, 2023

Hofman MA, Swaab DF (May 1992). "Seasonal changes in the suprachiasmatic nucleus of man". Neuroscience Letters. 139 (2): 257–260. doi:10.1016/0304-3940(92)90566-p. hdl:20.500.11755/44b0a214-7ffe-4a5d-b8e5-290354dd93f5. PMID 1608556. S2CID 22326141. Archived from the original on 20 November 2020. Retrieved 22 October 2020.

Tramontin AD, Brenowitz EA (June 2000). "Seasonal plasticity in the adult brain". Trends in Neurosciences. 23 (6): 251–8. doi:10.1016/s0166-2236(00)01558-7. PMID 10838594. S2CID 16888328.

Makris GD, Reutfors J, Larsson R, Isacsson G, Ösby U, Ekbom A, Ekselius L, Papadopoulos FC. Serotonergic medication enhances the association between suicide and sunshine. J Affect Disord. 2016 Jan 1;189:276-81. doi: 10.1016/j.jad.2015.09.056. Epub 2015 Oct 8. PMID: 26454332.

Lambert GW, Reid C, Kaye DM, Jennings GL, Esler MD. Effect of sunlight and season on serotonin turnover in the brain. Lancet.

2002 Dec 7;360(9348):1840-2. doi: 10.1016/s0140-6736(02)11737-5. PMID: 12480364

Gupta A, Sharma PK, Garg VK, Singh AK, Mondal SC. Role of serotonin in seasonal affective disorder. Eur Rev Med Pharmacol Sci. 2013 Jan;17(1):49-55. PMID: 23329523.

Sun L, Malén T, Tuisku J, Kaasinen V, Hietala JA, Rinne J, Nuutila P, Nummenmaa L. Seasonal variation in D2/3 dopamine receptor availability in the human brain. Eur J Nucl Med Mol Imaging. 2024 Sep;51(11):3284-3291. doi: 10.1007/s00259-024-06715-9. Epub 2024 May 11. PMID: 38730083; PMCID: PMC11369044.

Chapter 15

Living in Balance with Maharishi AyurVeda: Practical Therapies for Consciousness-Based Health by Robert Keith Wallace, PhD, Karin Pirc, MD, Julia Clarke, MS, MIU Press, 2023

Chapter 16

16 Super Biohacks for Longevity: Shortcuts to a Healthier, Happier, Longer Life by Robert Keith Wallace, PhD, Ted Wallace, MS, Samantha Wallace , Dharma Publications, 2023

Neurohacking for Online Learning: Study and Life Habits Optimized for your Personal Mind-Body Energy Stat by Robert Keith Wallace, PhD, Carol Paredes, MS, Dharma Publications, 2023

Chapter 17

Hamblin MR. Photobiomodulation for Alzheimer's Disease: Has the Light Dawned? Photonics. 2019 Sep;6(3):77. doi: 10.3390/photonics6030077. Epub 2019 Jul 4. PMID: 31363464; PMCID: PMC6664299.

Montazeri K, Farhadi M, Fekrazad R, Akbarnejad Z, Chaibakhsh S, Mahmoudian S. Transcranial photobiomodulation in the management of brain disorders. J Photochem Photobiol B. 2021 Aug;221:112207. doi: 10.1016/j.jphotobiol.2021.112207. Epub 2021 May 5. PMID: 34119804.

Do MTH. Melanopsin and the Intrinsically Photosensitive Retinal Ganglion Cells: Biophysics to Behavior. Neuron. 2019 Oct 23;104(2):205-226. doi: 10.1016/j.neuron.2019.07.016. PMID: 31647894; PMCID: PMC6944442.

Lazzerini Ospri L, Prusky G, Hattar S. Mood, the Circadian System, and Melanopsin Retinal Ganglion Cells. Annu Rev Neurosci. 2017 Jul 25;40:539-556. doi: 10.1146/annurev-neuro-072116-031324. Epub 2017 May 17. PMID: 28525301; PMCID: PMC5654534.

Barolet D, Christiaens F, Hamblin MR. Infrared and skin: Friend or foe. J Photochem Photobiol B. 2016 Feb;155:78-85. doi: 10.1016/j.jphotobiol.2015.12.014. Epub 2015 Dec 21. PMID: 26745730; PMCID: PMC4745411

Reiter RJ, Tan DX, Rosales-Corral S, Galano A, Zhou XJ, Xu B. Mitochondria: Central Organelles for Melatonin's Antioxidant and Anti-Aging Actions. Molecules. 2018 Feb 24;23(2):509. doi: 10.3390/molecules 23020509. PMID: 29495303; PMCID: PMC6017324.

Reiter RJ, Ma Q, Sharma R. Melatonin in Mitochondria: Mitigating Clear and Present Dangers. Physiology (Bethesda). 2020 Mar 1;35(2):86-95. doi: 10.1152/physiol.00034.2019. PMID: 32024428.

Melhuish Beaupre LM, Brown GM, Gonçalves VF, Kennedy JL. Melatonin's neuroprotective role in mitochondria and its potential as a biomarker in aging, cognition and psychiatric disorders. Transl Psychiatry. 2021 Jun 2;11(1):339. doi: 10.1038/s41398-021-01464-x. PMID: 34078880; PMCID: PMC8172874.

Reiter RJ, Sharma R, Pires de Campos Zuccari DA, de Almeida Chuffa LG, Manucha W, Rodriguez C. Melatonin synthesis in and uptake by mitochondria: implications for diseased cells with dysfunctional mitochondria. Future Med Chem. 2021 Feb;13(4):335-339. doi: 10.4155/fmc-2020-0326. Epub 2021 Jan 5. PMID: 33399498.

Engel KW, Khan I, Arany PR. Cell lineage responses to photobiomodulation therapy. J Biophotonics. 2016 Dec;9(11-12):1148-1156. doi:

10.1002/jbio.201600025. Epub 2016 Jul 8. PMID: 27392170.

Srivastava AK, Roy Choudhury S, Karmakar S. Near-Infrared Responsive Dopamine/Melatonin-Derived Nanocomposites Abrogating in Situ Amyloid β Nucleation, Propagation, and Ameliorate Neuronal Functions. ACS Appl Mater Interfaces. 2020 Feb 5;12(5):5658-5670. doi: 10.1021/acsami.9b22214. Epub 2020 Jan 27. PMID: 31986005.

Reiter RJ, Sharma R, Rosales-Corral S. Anti-Warburg Effect of Melatonin: A Proposed Mechanism to Explain its Inhibition of Multiple Diseases. Int J Mol Sci. 2021 Jan 14;22(2):764. doi: 10.3390/ijms22020764. PMID: 33466614; PMCID: PMC7828708.

Dr Andrew Huberman, Neurobiologicist and Associate Professor at Stanford talks about the value of sunlight: https://www.youtube.com/watch?v=yBjUR16AiBMD

Sansone RA, Sansone LA. Sunshine, serotonin, and skin: a partial explanation for seasonal patterns in psychopathology? Innov Clin Neurosci. 2013 Jul;10(7-8):20-4. PMID: 24062970; PMCID: PMC3779905.

Praschak-Rieder N, Willeit M, Wilson AA, et al. Seasonal variation in human brain serotonin transporter binding. Arch Gen Psychiatry. 2008;65:1072–1078.

Rosenthal NE, Sack DA, Gillin JC, et al. Seasonal affective disorder: a description of the syndrome and preliminary findings with light therapy. Arch Gen Psychiatry. 1984;41:72–80.

Tuunainen A, Kripke DF, Endo T. Light therapy for non-seasonal depression. Cochrane Database Syst Rev. 2004:CD004050.

Lieverse R, Van Someren EJW, Nielen MMA, et al. Bright light treatment in elderly patients with nonseasonal major depressive disorder: a randomized placebo-controlled trial. Arch Gen Psychiatry. 2011;68:61–70.

Cawley EI, Park S, aan het Rot M, Sancton K, Benkelfat C, Young SN, Boivin DB, Leyton M. Dopamine and light: dissecting effects on mood and motivational states in women with subsyndromal seasonal affective disorder. J Psychiatry Neurosci. 2013 Nov;38(6):388-97. doi: 10.1503/jpn.120181. PMID: 23735584; PMCID: PMC3819153.

Tsai HY, Chen KC, Yang YK, Chen PS, Yeh TL, Chiu NT, Lee IH. Sunshine-exposure variation of human striatal dopamine D(2)/D(3) receptor availability in healthy volunteers. Prog Neuropsychopharmacol Biol

Psychiatry. 2011 Jan 15;35(1):107-10. doi: 10.1016/j.pnpbp.2010.09.014. Epub 2010 Sep 26. PMID: 20875835.

Roy S, Field GD. Dopaminergic modulation of retinal processing from starlight to sunlight. J Pharmacol Sci. 2019 May;140(1):86-93. doi: 10.1016/j.jphs.2019.03.006. Epub 2019 May 4. PMID: 31109761.

Young SN. How to increase serotonin in the human brain without drugs. J Psychiatry Neurosci. 2007 Nov;32(6):394-9. PMID: 18043762; PMCID: PMC2077351.

Chapter 18

Living in Balance with Maharishi AyurVeda: Practical Therapies for Consciousness-Based Health by Robert Keith Wallace, PhD, Karin Pirc, MD, Julia Clarke, MS, MIU Press, 2023

The Rest And Repair Diet: Heal Your Gut, Improve Your Physical and Mental Health, and Lose Weight by Robert Keith Wallace, PhD, Samantha Wallace, Andrew Sternberg, MA Jim Davis, DO, and Alexis Farley, Dharma Publications, 2019

Puchalska P, Crawford PA. Multi-dimensional Roles of Ketone Bodies in Fuel Metabolism, Signaling, and Therapeutics. Cell Metab. 2017 Feb 7;25(2):262-284. doi: 10.1016/j.cmet.2016.12.022. PMID: 28178565; PMCID: PMC5313038.

Miriam, B et al. Added Sugars and Cardiovascular Disease Risk in Children: A Scientific Statement From the American Heart Association, Circulation. 2017 May 09; 135(19): e1017–e1034

Serena, G et al. The Role of Gluten in Celiac Disease and Type 1 Diabetes. Nutrients 2015 Aug 26;7(9):7143-62

Leonardi, GC et al., Ageing: from inflammation to cancer. Immunity and Ageing 2018; 15:1Fasano, A, Intestinal permeability and its regulation by zonulin: diagnosis and therapeutic implications. Clinical Gastroenterology and Hepatology 2012; 10,1096-100

Fasano, A. Zonulin, Regulation of tight junctions, and autoimmune diseases. Annals of the New York Academy of Sciences 2012; 1258(1):25-33

Chapter 19

Wallace, RK. The Microbiome in Health and Disease from the Perspective of Modern Medicine and Ayurveda. Medicina 2020; 56, 462.

Wallace, R.K. Ayurgenomics and Modern Medicine. Medicina 2020, 56, 661.

Gut Crisis: How Diet, Probiotics, and Friendly Bacteria Help You Lose Weight and Heal Your Body and Mind by Robert Keith Wallace, PhD, Samantha Wallace, Dharma Publications, 2017

Dale HF, Rasmussen SH, Asiller ÖÖ, Lied GA. Probiotics in Irritable Bowel Syndrome: An Up-to-Date Systematic Review. Nutrients. 2019 Sep 2;11(9):2048. doi: 10.3390/nu11092048. PMID: 31480656; PMCID:PMC6769995.

Chapter 20

Neurotransmitter Supplements
Selasi Attipoe, Stacey A. Zeno, Courtney Lee, Cindy Crawford, Raheleh Khorsan, Avi R. Walter, Patricia A. Deuster, Tyrosine for Mitigating Stress and Enhancing Performance in Healthy Adult Humans, a Rapid Evidence Assessment of the Literature, Military Medicine, Volume 180, Issue 7, July 2015, Pages 754–765, https://doi.org/10.7205/MILMED-D-14-00594

Ivanova Stojcheva E, Quintela JC. The Effectiveness of Rhodiola rosea L. Preparations in Alleviating Various Aspects of Life-Stress Symptoms and Stress-Induced Conditions-Encouraging Clinical Evidence. Molecules. 2022 Jun 17;27(12):3902. doi: 10.3390/molecules27123902. PMID: 35745023; PMCID: PMC9228580.

Blum K, Chen TJ, Meshkin B, Waite RL, Downs BW, Blum SH, Mengucci JF, Arcuri V, Braverman ER, Palomo T. Manipulation of catechol-O-methyl-transferase (COMT) activity to influence the attenuation of substance seeking behavior, a subtype of Reward Deficiency Syndrome (RDS), is dependent upon gene polymorphisms: a hypothesis.

Med Hypotheses. 2007;69(5):1054-60. doi: 10.1016/j.mehy.2006.12.062. Epub 2007 Apr 30. PMID: 17467918.

Lampariello LR, Cortelazzo A, Guerranti R, Sticozzi C, Valacchi G. The Magic Velvet Bean of Mucuna pruriens. J Tradit Complement Med. 2012 Oct;2(4):331-9. doi: 10.1016/s2225-4110(16)30119-5. PMID: 24716148; PMCID: PMC3942911.

Pulikkalpura H, Kurup R, Mathew PJ, Baby S. Levodopa in Mucuna pruriens and its degradation. Sci Rep. 2015 Jun 9;5:11078. doi: 10.1038/srep11078. PMID: 26058043; PMCID: PMC4460905.

Kikuchi AM, Tanabe A, Iwahori Y. A systematic review of the effect of L-tryptophan supplementation on mood and emotional functioning. J Diet Suppl. 2021;18(3):316-333. doi: 10.1080/19390211.2020.1746725. Epub 2020 Apr 10. PMID: 32272859.

Maffei ME. 5-Hydroxytryptophan (5-HTP): Natural Occurrence, Analysis, Biosynthesis, Biotechnology, Physiology and Toxicology. Int J Mol Sci. 2020 Dec 26;22(1):181. doi: 10.3390/ijms22010181. PMID: 33375373; PMCID: PMC7796270.

Zhao X, Zhang H, Wu Y, Yu C. The efficacy and safety of St. John's wort extract in depression therapy compared to SSRIs in adults: A meta-analysis of randomized clinical trials. Adv Clin Exp Med. 2023 Feb;32(2):151-161. doi: 10.17219/acem/152942. PMID: 36226689.

Linde K, Berner MM, Kriston L. St John's wort for major depression. Cochrane Database Syst Rev. 2008 Oct 08;2008(4):CD000448. [

Rapaport MH, Nierenberg AA, Howland R, Dording C, Schettler PJ, Mischoulon D. The treatment of minor depression with St. John's Wort or citalopram: failure to show benefit over placebo. J Psychiatr Res. 2011 Jul;45(7):931-41

Pascale RM, Simile MM, Calvisi DF, Feo CF, Feo F. S-Adenosylmethionine: From the Discovery of Its Inhibition of Tumorigenesis to Its Use as a Therapeutic Agent. Cells. 2022 Jan 25;11(3):409. doi: 10.3390/cells11030409. PMID: 35159219; PMCID: PMC8834208.

Galizia, I; Oldani, L; Macritchie, K; Amari, E; Dougall, D; Jones, TN; Lam, RW; Massei, GJ; Yatham, LN; Young, AH (10 October 2016). "S-Adenosyl methionine (SAMe) for depression in adults". The Cochrane Database of Systematic Reviews. 2016 (10): CD011286.

doi:10.1002/14651858.CD011286.pub2. PMC 6457972. PMID 27727432

Tamura Y, Takata K, Matsubara K, Kataoka Y. Alpha-Glycerylphosphorylcholine Increases Motivation in Healthy Volunteers: A Single-Blind, Randomized, Placebo-Controlled Human Study. Nutrients. 2021 Jun 18;13(6):2091. doi: 10.3390/nu13062091. PMID: 34207484; PMCID: PMC8235064.

Qian ZM, Ke Y. Huperzine A: Is it an Effective Disease-Modifying Drug for Alzheimer's Disease? Front Aging Neurosci. 2014 Aug 19;6:216. doi: 10.3389/fnagi.2014.00216. PMID: 25191267; PMCID: PMC4137276.

Friedli MJ, Inestrosa NC. Huperzine A and Its Neuroprotective Molecular Signaling in Alzheimer's Disease. Molecules. 2021 Oct 29;26(21):6531. doi: 10.3390/molecules26216531. PMID: 34770940; PMCID: PMC8587556.

Liu M, Li T, Liang H, Zhong P. Herbal medicines in Alzheimer's disease and the involvement of gut microbiota. Front Pharmacol. 2024 Jul 16;15:1416502. doi: 10.3389/fphar.2024.1416502. PMID: 39081953; PMCID: PMC11286407.

Pervin M, Unno K, Takagaki A, Isemura M, Nakamura Y. Function of Green Tea Catechins in the Brain: Epigallocatechin Gallate and its Metabolites. Int J Mol Sci. 2019 Jul 25;20(15):3630. doi: 10.3390/ijms20153630. PMID: 31349535; PMCID: PMC6696481.

Ayurveda Supplements

Sharma H, Wallace RK. Ayurveda and Epigenetics. Medicina (Kaunas). 2020 Dec 11;56(12):687. doi: 10.3390/medicina56120687. PMID: 33322263; PMCID: PMC7763202.

Peterson CT, Denniston K, Chopra D. Therapeutic Uses of Triphala in Ayurvedic Medicine. J Altern Complement Med. 2017 Aug;23(8):607-614. doi: 10.1089/acm.2017.0083. Epub 2017 Jul 11. PMID: 28696777; PMCID: PMC5567597.

Baliga MS, et al. Scientific validation of the ethnomedicinal properties of the Ayurvedic drug Triphala: A review. Chin J Integr Med 2012;18:946–954

Wang W, Ige OO, Ding Y, He M, Long P, Wang S, Zhang Y, Wen X.

Insights into the potential benefits of triphala polyphenols toward the promotion of resilience against stress-induced depression and cognitive impairment. Curr Res Food Sci. 2023 Jun 2;6:100527. doi: 10.1016/j. crfs.2023.100527. PMID: 37377497; PMCID: PMC10291000.

Majeed M, Nagabhushanam K, Murali A, Vishwanathan DT, Mamidala RV, Mundkur L. A Standardized Withania somnifera (Linn.) Root Extract with Piperine Alleviates the Symptoms of Anxiety and Depression by Increasing Serotonin Levels: A Double-Blind, Randomized, Placebo-Controlled Study. J Integr Complement Med. 2024 May;30(5):459-468. doi: 10.1089/jicm.2023.0279. Epub 2023 Oct 25. PMID: 37878284.

Majeed M, Nagabhushanam K, Mundkur L. A standardized Ashwagandha root extract alleviates stress, anxiety, and improves quality of life in healthy adults by modulating stress hormones: Results from a randomized, double-blind, placebo-controlled study. Medicine (Baltimore). 2023 Oct 13;102(41):e35521. doi: 10.1097/MD.0000000000035521. PMID: 37832082; PMCID: PMC10578737.

Speers AB, Cabey KA, Soumyanath A, Wright KM. Effects of **Withania somnifera** (Ashwagandha) on Stress and the Stress-Related Neuropsychiatric Disorders Anxiety, Depression, and Insomnia. Curr Neuropharmacol. 2021;19(9):1468-1495. doi: 10.2174/1570159X19666621071215

1556. PMID: 34254920; PMCID: PMC8762185.

Lopresti AL, Smith SJ, Malvi H, Kodgule R. An investigation into the stress-relieving and pharmacological actions of an ashwagandha (Withania somnifera) extract: A randomized, double-blind, placebo-controlled study. Medicine (Baltimore). 2019 Sep;98(37):e17186. doi: 10.1097/MD.0000000000017186. PMID: 31517876; PMCID: PMC6750292.

Nemetchek MD, Stierle AA, Stierle DB, Lurie DI. The Ayurvedic plant Bacopa monnieri inhibits inflammatory pathways in the brain. J Ethnopharmacol. 2017 Feb 2;197:92-100. doi: 10.1016/j.jep.2016.07.073. Epub 2016 Jul 26. PMID: 27473605; PMCID: PMC5269610

Williams R, Münch G, Gyengesi E, Bennett L. Bacopa monnieri (L.) exerts anti-inflammatory effects on cells of the innate immune system in vitro. Food Funct. 2014 Mar;5(3):517-20. doi: 10.1039/c3fo60467e. PMID: 24452710.

Stough C, Lloyd J, Clarke J, Downey LA, Hutchison CW, Rodgers T, Nathan PJ. The chronic effects of an extract of Bacopa monniera (Brahmi) on cognitive function in healthy human subjects. Psychopharmacology (Berl). 2001 Aug;156(4):481-4. doi: 10.1007/s002130100815. Erratum in: Psychopharmacology (Berl). 2015 Jul;232(13):2427. Dosage error in article text. PMID: 11498727.

Peth-Nui T, Wattanathorn J, Muchimapura S, Tong-Un T, Piyavhatkul N, Rangseekajee P, IngkaTinan K, Vittaya-Areekul S. Effects of 12-Week Bacopa monnieri Consumption on Attention, Cognitive Processing, Working Memory, and Functions of Both Cholinergic and Monoaminergic Systems in Healthy Elderly Volunteers. Evid Based Complement Alternat Med. 2012;2012:606424. doi: 10.1155/2012/606424. Epub 2012 Dec 18. PMID: 23320031; PMCID: PMC3537209.

Rai D, Bhatia G, Palit G, Pal R, Singh S, Singh HK. Adaptogenic effect of Bacopa monniera (Brahmi). Pharmacol Biochem Behav. 2003 Jul;75(4):823-30. doi: 10.1016/s0091-3057(03)00156-4. PMID: 12957224.

Benson S, Downey LA, Stough C, Wetherell M, Zangara A, Scholey A. An acute, double-blind, placebo-controlled cross-over study of 320 mg and 640 mg doses of Bacopa monnieri (CDRI 08) on multitasking stress reactivity and mood. Phytother Res. 2014 Apr;28(4):551-9. doi: 10.1002/ptr.5029. Epub 2013 Jun 21. PMID: 23788517.

Calabrese C, Gregory WL, Leo M, Kraemer D, Bone K, Oken B. Effects of a standardized Bacopa monnieri extract on cognitive performance, anxiety, and depression in the elderly: a randomized, double-blind, placebo-controlled trial. J Altern Complement Med. 2008 Jul;14(6):707-13. doi: 10.1089/acm.2008.0018. PMID: 18611150; PMCID: PMC3153866.

Balkrishna A, Thakur P, Varshney A. Phytochemical Profile, Pharmacological Attributes and Medicinal Properties of Convolvulus prostratus - A Cognitive Enhancer Herb for the Management of Neurodegenerative Etiologies. Front Pharmacol. 2020 Mar 3;11:171. doi: 10.3389/fphar.2020.00171. PMID: 32194410; PMCID: PMC7063970.

Mukerjee N, Al-Khafaji K, Maitra S, Suhail Wadi J, Sachdeva P, Ghosh A, et al. Recognizing novel drugs against Keap1 in AD using machine learning grounded computational studies. Front Mol Neurosci. 2022;15:1036552.

Francis PT, Plamer AM, Anape M, et al. The cholinergic hypothesis of

Alzheimer's dieases: a review of progress. J Neurol Neurosurg Psychiatry. 1999;66(2):137–47.

Tomeh MA, Hadianamrei R, Zhao X. A Review of Curcumin and Its Derivatives as Anticancer Agents. Int J Mol Sci. 2019 Feb 27;20(5):1033. doi: 10.3390/ijms20051033. PMID: 30818786; PMCID: PMC6429287.

Salehi B, Stojanović-Radić Z, Matejić J, Sharifi-Rad M, Anil Kumar NV, Martins N, Sharifi-Rad J. The therapeutic potential of curcumin: A review of clinical trials. Eur J Med Chem. 2019 Feb 1;163:527-545. doi: 10.1016/j.ejmech.2018.12.016. Epub 2018 Dec 7. PMID: 30553144.

Lang A, Salomon N, Wu JC, Kopylov U, Lahat A, HarNoy O, et al. Curcumin in combination with mesalamine induces remission in patients with mild to moderate ulcerative colitis in a randomized controlled trial. Clin Gastroenterol Hepatol 2015;13:14449.e1.

Sudheeran SP, Jacob D, Mulakal JN, Nair GG, Maliakel A, Maliakel B, et al. Safety, tolerance, and enhanced efficacy of a bioavailable formulation of curcumin with fenugreek dietary fiber on occupational stress: a randomized, doubleblind, placebocontrolled pilot study. J Clin Psychopharmacol 2016;36:23643.

Aggarwal BB, Harikumar KB. Potential therapeutic effects of curcumin, the anti-inflammatory agent, against neurodegenerative, cardiovascular, pulmonary, metabolic, autoimmune and neoplastic Int J Biochem Cell Biol 2009;41:4059.

Venigalla M, Sonego S, Gyengesi E, Sharman MJ, Münch G. Novel promising therapeutics against chronic neuroinflammation and neurodegeneration in Alzheimer's disease. Neurochem Int 2016;95:6374.

Nelson KM, Dahlin JL, Bisson J, Graham J, Pauli GF, Walters MA. The Essential Medicinal Chemistry of Curcumin. J Med Chem. 2017 Mar 9;60(5):1620-1637. doi: 10.1021/acs.jmedchem.6b00975. Epub 2017 Jan 11. PMID: 28074653; PMCID: PMC5346970.

General Supplements
Moyer VA, U. S. Preventive Services Task Force. Vitamin, mineral, and multivitamin supplements for the primary prevention of cardiovascular disease and cancer: U.S. Preventive services Task Force recommendation statement. Ann Intern Med. 2014;160(8):558–64. PMID: 24566474.

10.7326/M14-0198

Fairfield KM. Vitamin supplementation in disease prevention. Seres D, ed. Waltham, MA: UpToDate. http://www.uptodate.com. Accessed December 7, 2018: 2020.

National Center for Complementary and Integrative Health, National Institutes of Health. Vitamins and Minerals. https://nccih.nih.gov/health/vitamins. Accessed: July 31, 2020.

Papadopol V, Nechifor M. Magnesium in neuroses and neuroticism. In: Vink R, Nechifor M, editors. Magnesium in the Central Nervous System [Internet]. Adelaide (AU): University of Adelaide Press; 2011. Available from: https://www.ncbi.nlm.nih.gov/books/NBK507254/

DiNicolantonio JJ, O'Keefe JH. The Importance of Marine Omega-3s for Brain Development and the Prevention and Treatment of Behavior, Mood, and Other Brain Disorders. Nutrients. 2020 Aug 4;12(8):2333. doi: 10.3390/nu12082333. PMID: 32759851; PMCID: PMC7468918.

Bischoff-Ferrari HA, Vellas B, Rizzoli R, Kressig RW, da Silva JAP, Blauth M, Felson DT, McCloskey EV, Watzl B, Hofbauer LC, Felsenberg D, Willett WC, Dawson-Hughes B, Manson JE, Siebert U, Theiler R, Staehelin HB, de Godoi Rezende Costa Molino C, Chocano-Bedoya PO, Abderhalden LA, Egli A, Kanis JA, Orav EJ; DO-HEALTH Research Group. Effect of Vitamin D Supplementation, Omega-3 Fatty Acid Supplementation, or a Strength-Training Exercise Program on Clinical Outcomes in Older Adults: The DO-HEALTH Randomized Clinical Trial. JAMA. 2020 Nov 10;324(18):1855-1868. doi: 10.1001/jama.2020.16909. PMID: 33170239; PMCID: PMC7656284.

Rauch, B.; Schiele, R.; Schneider, S.; Diller, F.; Victor, N.; Gohlke, H.; Gottwik, M.; Steinbeck, G.; Del Castillo, U.; Sack, R.; et al. OMEGA, a randomized, placebo-controlled trial to test the effect of highly purified omega-3 fatty acids on top of modern guideline-adjusted therapy after myocardial infarction. Circulation 2010, 122, 2152–2159.

McCarty, M.F.; DiNicolantonio, J.J.; Lavie, C.J.; O'Keefe, J.H. Omega-3 and prostate cancer: Examining the pertinent evidence. Mayo Clin. Proc. 2014, 89, 444–450.

DiNicolantonio, J.J.; Mccarty, M.F.; Lavie, C.J.; O'Keefe, J.H. Do omega-3 fatty acids cause prostate cancer? MO Med. 2013,110, 293–294.

Hu Y, Hu FB, Manson JE. Marine Omega-3 Supplementation and Cardiovascular Disease: An Updated Meta-Analysis of 13 Randomized Controlled Trials Involving 127 477 Participants. J Am Heart Assoc. 2019 Oct;8(19):e013543. doi: 10.1161/JAHA.119.013543. Epub 2019 Sep 30. PMID: 31567003; PMCID: PMC6806028.

Pravst I, Rodríguez Aguilera JC, Cortes Rodriguez AB, Jazbar J, Locatelli I, Hristov H, Žmitek K. Comparative Bioavailability of Different Coenzyme Q10 Formulations in Healthy Elderly Individuals. Nutrients. 2020 Mar 16;12(3):784. doi: 10.3390/nu12030784. PMID: 32188111; PMCID: PMC7146408.

Chapter 21

Living in Balance with Maharishi AyurVeda by Robert Keith Wallace, PhD, Karin Pirc, MD, Julia Clarke, MS, MIU Press, 2023, in press

Schneider, RH, et al., Health Promotion with a Traditional System of Natural Health Care: Maharishi Ayurveda, 1990, Journal of Social Behavior and Personality, 5(3): 1-27

Waldschutz, R. Physiological and Psychological Changes Associated with Ayurvedic Purification Treatment, 1988, Erfahrungsheilkunde—Acta Medico Empirica—Zeitschrift fur die drztliche Praxis, 2: 720-729

Herron RE, Fagan JB. Lipophil-mediated reduction of toxicants in humans: an evaluation of an ayurvedic detoxification procedure. Altern Ther Health Med. 2002 Sep-Oct;8(5):40-51. PMID: 12233802.

The Brain Maker: The Power of Gut Microbes to Heal and Protect Your Brain for Life by Dr. David Perlmutter, Little, Brown Spark, 2015

Chapter 22

Holst SC, Landolt HP. Sleep-Wake Neurochemistry. Sleep Med Clin. 2018 Jun;13(2):137-146. doi: 10.1016/j.jsmc.2018.03.002. PMID: 29759265.

Vashadze ShV. [Insomnia, serotonin and depression]. Georgian Med News. 2007 Sep;(150):22-4. Russian. PMID: 17984558. Arendt J.

Melatonin: Countering Chaotic Time Cues. Front Endocrinol (Lausanne). 2019 Jul 16;10:391. doi: 10.3389/fendo.2019.00391. PMID: 31379733; PMCID: PMC6646716.

Poza JJ, Pujol M, Ortega-Albás JJ, Romero O; Insomnia Study Group of the Spanish Sleep Society (SES). Melatonin in sleep disorders. Neurologia (Engl Ed). 2022 Sep;37(7):575-585. doi: 10.1016/j.nrleng.2018.08.004. Epub 2020 Sep 18. PMID: 36064286.

Bueno APR, Savi FM, Alves IA, Bandeira VAC. Regulatory aspects and evidences of melatonin use for sleep disorders and insomnia: an integrative review. Arq Neuropsiquiatr. 2021 Aug;79(8):732-742. doi: 10.1590/0004-282X-ANP-2020-0379. PMID: 34550191.

Besag FMC, Vasey MJ, Lao KSJ, Wong ICK. Adverse Events Associated with Melatonin for the Treatment of Primary or Secondary Sleep Disorders: A Systematic Review. CNS Drugs. 2019 Dec;33(12):1167-1186. doi: 10.1007/s40263-019-00680-w. PMID: 31722088.

Reiter RJ, Ma Q, Sharma R. Melatonin in Mitochondria: Mitigating Clear and Present Dangers. Physiology (Bethesda). 2020 Mar 1;35(2):86-95. doi: 10.1152/physiol.00034.2019. PMID: 32024428.

Melhuish Beaupre LM, Brown GM, Gonçalves VF, Kennedy JL. Melatonin's neuroprotective role in mitochondria and its potential as a biomarker in aging, cognition and psychiatric disorders. Transl Psychiatry. 2021 Jun 2;11(1):339.

Li T, Jiang S, Han M, Yang Z, Lv J, Deng C, Reiter RJ, Yang Y. Exogenous melatonin as a treatment for secondary sleep disorders: A systematic review and meta-analysis. Front Neuroendocrinol. 2019 Jan;52:22-28. doi: 10.1016/j.yfrne.2018.06.004. Epub 2018 Jun 15. PMID: 29908879.

Foley HM, Steel AE. Adverse events associated with oral administration of melatonin: A critical systematic review of clinical evidence. Complement Ther Med. 2019 Feb;42:65-81. doi: 10.1016/j.ctim.2018.11.003. Epub 2018 Nov 3. PMID: 30670284.

Scholtens RM, van Munster BC, van Kempen MF, de Rooij SE. Physiological melatonin levels in healthy older people: A systematic review. J Psychosom Res. 2016 Jul;86:20-7. doi: 10.1016/j.jpsychores.2016.05.005. Epub 2016 May 10. PMID: 27302542.

Culpepper L, Wingertzahn MA. Over-the-Counter Agents for the

Treatment of Occasional Disturbed Sleep or Transient Insomnia: A Systematic Review of Efficacy and Safety. Prim Care Companion CNS Disord. 2015 Dec 31;17(6):10.4088/PCC.15r01798. doi: 10.4088/ PCC.15r01798. PMID: 27057416; PMCID: PMC4805417.

Zare Elmi HK, Gholami M, Saki M, Ebrahimzadeh F. Efficacy of Valerian Extract on Sleep Quality after Coronary Artery bypass Graft Surgery: A Triple-Blind Randomized Controlled Trial. Chin J Integr Med. 2021 Jan;27(1):7-15. doi: 10.1007/s11655-020-2727-1. Epub 2021 Jan 8. PMID: 33420602.

Murray BJ, Cowen PJ, Sharpley AL. The effect of Li 1370, extract of Ginkgo biloba, on REM sleep in humans. Pharmacopsychiatry. 2001 Jul;34(4):155-7. doi: 10.1055/s-2001-15876. PMID: 11518478.

Djokic G, Vojvodić P, Korcok D, Agic A, Rankovic A, Djordjevic V, Vojvodic A, Vlaskovic-Jovicevic T, Peric-Hajzler Z, Matovic D, Vojvodic J, Sijan G, Wollina U, Tirant M, Thuong NV, Fioranelli M, Lotti T. The Effects of Magnesium - Melatonin - Vit B Complex Supplementation in Treatment of Insomnia. Open Access Maced J Med Sci. 2019 Aug 30;7(18):3101-3105. doi: 10.3889/oamjms.2019.771. PMID: 31850132; PMCID: PMC6910806.

Sutanto CN, Loh WW, Kim JE. The impact of tryptophan supplementation on sleep quality: a systematic review, meta-analysis, and meta-regression. Nutr Rev. 2022 Jan 10;80(2):306-316. doi: 10.1093/nutrit/ nuab027. PMID: 33942088.

Dasdelen MF, Er S, Kaplan B, Celik S, Beker MC, Orhan C, Tuzcu M, Sahin N, Mamedova H, Sylla S, Komorowski J, Ojalvo SP, Sahin K, Kilic E. A Novel Theanine Complex, Mg-L-Theanine Improves Sleep Quality via Regulating Brain Electrochemical Activity. Front Nutr. 2022 Apr 5;9:874254. doi: 10.3389/fnut.2022.874254. PMID: 35449538; PMCID: PMC9017334.

Fetveit A, Skjerve A, Bjorvatn B. Bright light treatment improves sleep in institutionalised elderly-an open trial. Int J Geriatr Psychiatry. 2003 Jun;18(6):520-6. doi: 10.1002/gps.852. PMID: 12789673.

Higuchi S, Motohashi Y, Liu Y, Maeda A. Effects of playing a computer game using a bright display on presleep physiological variables, sleep latency, slow wave sleep and REM sleep. J Sleep Res. 2005 Sep;14(3):267-73. doi: 10.1111/j.1365-2869.2005.00463.x. PMID: 16120101.

Kanda K, Tochihara Y, Ohnaka T. Bathing before sleep in the young and in the elderly. Eur J Appl Physiol Occup Physiol. 1999 Jul;80(2):71-5. doi: 10.1007/s004210050560. PMID: 10408315.

Youngstedt SD, Kripke DF, Elliott JA. Is sleep disturbed by vigorous late-night exercise? Med Sci Sports Exerc. 1999 Jun;31(6):864-9. doi: 10.1097/00005768-199906000-00015. PMID: 10378914.

Chapter 23

Marques A, Marconcin P, Werneck AO, Ferrari G, Gouveia ÉR, Kliegel M, Peralta M, Ihle A. Bidirectional Association between Physical Activity and Dopamine Across Adulthood-A Systematic Review. Brain Sci. 2021 Jun 23;11(7):829. doi: 10.3390/brainsci11070829. PMID: 34201523; PMCID: PMC8301978.

Lee DH, Rezende LFM, Joh HK, Keum N, Ferrari G, Rey-Lopez JP, Rimm EB, Tabung FK, Giovannucci EL. Long-Term Leisure-Time Physical Activity Intensity and All-Cause and Cause-Specific Mortality: A Prospective Cohort of US Adults. Circulation. 2022 Aug 16;146(7):523-534. doi: 10.1161/CIRCULATIONAHA.121.058162. Epub 2022 Jul 25. PMID: 35876019; PMCID: PMC9378548.

Mu X, Liu S, Fu M, Luo M, Ding D, Chen L, Yu K. Associations of physical activity intensity with incident cardiovascular diseases and mortality among 366,566 UK adults. Int J Behav Nutr Phys Act. 2022 Dec 13;19(1):151. doi: 10.1186/s12966-022-01393-y. PMID: 36514169; PMCID: PMC9745930.

Wang Y, Nie J, Ferrari G, Rey-Lopez JP, Rezende LFM. Association of Physical Activity Intensity With Mortality: A National Cohort Study of 403 681 US Adults. JAMA Intern Med. 2021 Feb 1;181(2):203-211. doi: 10.1001/jAmainternmed.2020.6331. PMID: 33226432; PMCID: PMC7684516.

Sanders LMJ, Hortobágyi T, Karssemeijer EGA, Van der Zee EA, Scherder EJA, van Heuvelen MJG. Effects of low- and high-intensity physical exercise on physical and cognitive function in older persons with dementia: a randomized controlled trial. Alzheimers Res

Ther. 2020 Mar 19;12(1):28. doi: 10.1186/s13195-020-00597-3. PMID: 32192537; PMCID: PMC7082953.

Aguib Y, Al Suwaidi J. The Copenhagen City Heart Study (Øster-broundersøgelsen). Glob Cardiol Sci Pract. 2015 Oct 9;2015(3):33. doi: 10.5339/gcsp.2015.33. PMID: 26779513; PMCID: PMC4625209.

Atakan MM, Li Y, Koşar ŞN, Turnagöl HH, Yan X. Evidence-Based Effects of High-Intensity Interval Training on Exercise Capacity and Health: A Review with Historical Perspective. Int J Environ Res Public Health. 2021 Jul 5;18(13):7201. doi: 10.3390/ijerph18137201. PMID: 34281138; PMCID: PMC8294064.

Booth, FW; Roberts, C.K; Laye, M.J. Lack of exercise is a major cause of chronic diseases. Compr. Physiol. 2012, 2, 1143–1211

Hallal, PC. Andersen, L.B.; Bull, F.C.; Guthold, R.; Haskell, W.; Ekelund, U. Global physical activity levels: Surveillance progress, pitfalls, and prospects. Lancet 2012, 380, 247–257.

Bull, FC; Al-Ansari, SS; Biddle, S; Borodulin, K; Buman, MP; Cardon, G.; Carty, C.; Chaput, JP.; Chastin, S.; Chou, R.; et al. World Health Organization 2020 guidelines on physical activity and sedentary behaviour. Br. J. Sports Med. 2020, 54, 1451–1462.

Paluch AE, Gabriel KP, Fulton JE, et al. Steps per Day and All-Cause Mortality in Middle-aged Adults in the Coronary Artery Risk Development in Young Adults Study. **JAMA Netw Open.** 2021;4(9):e2124516. doi:10.1001/jAmanetworkopen.2021.24516

Sleiman SF, Henry J, Al-Haddad R, El Hayek L, Abou Haidar E, Stringer T, Ulja D, Karuppagounder SS, Holson EB, Ratan RR, Tinan I, Chao MV. Exercise promotes the expression of brain derived neurotrophic factor (BDNF) through the action of the ketone body β-hydroxybutyrate. Elife. 2016 Jun 2;5:e15092. doi: 10.7554/eLife.15092. PMID: 27253067; PMCID: PMC4915811.

Cooney GM, et al. Exercise for depression. JAMA. 2014;311:2432.

Peterson DM. The benefits and risks of exercise. https://www.uptodate.com/contents/search. Accessed Sept. 15, 2017.

Greer TL, et al. Improvements in psychosocial functioning and health-related quality of life following exercise augmentation in patients with treatment response but nonremitted major depressive disorder:

Results from the TREAD study. Depression and Anxiety. 2016;33:870.

Schuch FB, et al. Exercise as treatment for depression: A meta-analysis adjusting for publication bias. Journal of Psychiatric Research. 2016;77:42.

Zschucke E, et al. Exercise and physical activity in mental disorders: Clinical and experimental evidence. Journal of Preventive Medicine and Public Health. 2013;46:512.

Anderson E, et al. Effects of exercise and physical activity on anxiety. Frontiers in Psychiatry. 2013;4:1.

Isaac AR, Lima-Filho RAS, Lourenco MV. How does the skeletal muscle communicate with the brain in health and disease? Neuropharmacology. 2021 Oct 1;197:108744. doi: 10.1016/j.neuropharm.2021.108744.

Epub 2021 Aug 5. PMID: 34363812

Chapter 24

R P, Kumar AP, Dhamodhini K S, Venugopal V, Silambanan S, K M, Shah P. Role of yoga in stress management and implications in major depression disorder. J Ayurveda Integr Med. 2023 Sep-Oct;14(5):100767. doi: 10.1016/j.jaim.2023.100767. Epub 2023 Sep 21. PMID: 37741161; PMCID: PMC10520539

Lim S.-A., Cheong K.-J. Regular yoga practice improves antioxidant status, immune function, and stress hormone releases in young healthy people: a randomized, double-blind, controlled pilot study. J Alternative Compl Med. 2015;21(9):530–538. doi: 10.1089/acm.2014.0044

Estevao C. The role of yoga in inflammatory markers. Brain Behav Immun Health. 2022 Feb 1;20:100421. doi: 10.1016/j.bbih.2022.100421. PMID: 35199049; PMCID: PMC8842003.

Saeed SA, Cunningham K, Bloch RM. Depression and Anxiety Disorders: Benefits of Exercise, Yoga, and Meditation. Am Fam Physician. 2019 May 15;99(10):620-627. PMID: 31083878.

Wang WL, Chen KH, Pan YC, Yang SN, Chan YY. The effect of yoga on sleep quality and insomnia in women with sleep problems: a systematic review and meta-analysis. BMC Psychiatry. 2020 May 1;20(1):195. doi:

10.1186/s12888-020-02566-4. PMID: 32357858; PMCID: PMC7193366.

Groessl EJ, Liu L, Chang DG, Wetherell JL, Bormann JE, Atkinson JH, Baxi S, Schmalzl L. Yoga for Military Veterans with Chronic Low Back Pain: A Randomized Clinical Trial. Am J Prev Med. 2017 Nov;53(5):599-608. doi: 10.1016/j.amepre.2017.05.019. Epub 2017 Jul 20. PMID: 28735778; PMCID: PMC6399016.

Chapter 25

Ma X, Yue ZQ, Gong ZQ, Zhang H, Duan NY, Shi YT, Wei GX, Li YF. The Effect of Diaphragmatic Breathing on Attention, Negative Affect and Stress in Healthy Adults. Front Psychol. 2017 Jun 6;8:874. doi: 10.3389/fpsyg.2017.00874. PMID: 28626434; PMCID: PMC5455070.

Kressin, N. A., Nielsen, A. M., Laravuso, R. B., & Bisgard, G. E. (1984). RESPIRATORY EFFECTS OF DOMPERIDONE - PERIPHERAL DOPAMINE ANTAGONIST. Anesthesiology, 61(Supplement), A468. doi:10.1097/00000542-198409001-00468

Hopper SI, Murray SL, Ferrara LR, Singleton JK. Effectiveness of diaphragmatic breathing for reducing physiological and psychological stress in adults: a quantitative systematic review. JBI Database System Rev Implement Rep. 2019 Sep;17(9):1855-1876. doi: 10.11124/JBIS-RIR-2017-003848. PMID: 31436595.

Hamasaki H. Effects of Diaphragmatic Breathing on Health: A Narrative Review. Medicines (Basel). 2020 Oct 15;7(10):65. doi: 10.3390/medicines7100065. PMID: 33076360; PMCID: PMC7602530.

Jerath R., Crawford M.W., Barnes V.A., Harden K. Self-regulation of breathing as a primary treatment for anxiety. Appl. Psychophysiol. Biofeedback. 2015;40:107–115. doi: 10.1007/s10484-015-9279-8

Fincham, G.W., Strauss, C., Montero-Marin, J. et al. Effect of breathwork on stress and mental health: A meta-analysis of randomised-controlled trials. Sci Rep 13, 432 (2023). https://doi.org/10.1038/s41598-022-27247-y

Tainio M, Jovanovic Andersen Z, Nieuwenhuijsen MJ, Hu L, de Nazelle A, An R, Garcia LMT, Goenka S, Zapata-Diomedi B, Bull F, Sá TH. Air pollution, physical activity and health: A mapping review of the evidence.

Environ Int. 2021 Feb;147:105954. doi: 10.1016/j.envint.2020.105954. Epub 2020 Dec 19. PMID: 33352412; PMCID: PMC7816214.

Srinivasan TM. Pranayama and brain correlates. Anc Sci Life. 1991 Jul;11(1-2):2-6. PMID: 22556548; PMCID: PMC3336588.

Stancák A Jr, Pfeffer D, Hrudová L, Sovka P, Dostálek C. Electroencephalographic correlates of paced breathing. Neuroreport. 1993 Jun;4(6):723-6. doi: 10.1097/00001756-199306000-00031. PMID: 8347815.

Brennan SE, McDonald S, Murano M, McKenzie JE. Effectiveness of aromatherapy for prevention or treatment of disease, medical or preclinical conditions, and injury: protocol for a systematic review and meta-analysis. Syst Rev. 2022 Jul 26;11(1):148. doi: 10.1186/s13643-022-02015-1. PMID: 35883155; PMCID: PMC9317467.

Chapter 26

Yankouskaya A, Williamson R, Stacey C, Totman JJ, Massey H. Short-Term Head-Out Whole-Body Cold-Water Immersion Facilitates Positive Affect and Increases Interaction between Large-Scale Brain Networks. Biology (Basel). 2023 Jan 29;12(2):211. doi: 10.3390/biology12020211. PMID: 36829490; PMCID: PMC9953392.

Hirvonen J., Lindeman S., Joukamaa M., Huttunen P. Plasma catecholamines, serotonin and their metabolites and beta-endorphin of winter swimmers during one winter. Possible correlations to psychological traits. Int. J. Circumpolar Health. 2002;61:363–372. doi: 10.3402/ijch.v61i4.17494.

Esperland D, de Weerd L, Mercer JB. Health effects of voluntary exposure to cold water: a continuing subject of debate. Int J Circumpolar Health. 2022 Dec;81(1):2111789. doi: 10.1080/22423982.2022.2111789. PMID: 36137565; PMCID: PMC9518606.

Lorenzo I, Serra-Prat M, Yébenes JC. The Role of Water Homeostasis in Muscle Function and Frailty: A Review. Nutrients. 2019 Aug 9;11(8):1857. doi: 10.3390/nu11081857. PMID: 31405072; PMCID: PMC6723611.

Bondy SC, Campbell A. Water Quality and Brain Function. Int J Environ Res Public Health. 2017 Dec 21;15(1):2. doi: 10.3390/

ijerph15010002. PMID: 29267198; PMCID: PMC5800103. Esperland D, de Weerd L, Mercer JB. Health effects of voluntary exposure to cold water: a continuing subject of debate. Int J Circumpolar Health. 2022 Dec;81(1):2111789. doi: 10.1080/22423982.2022.2111789. PMID: 36137565; PMCID: PMC9518606.

Lorenzo I, Serra-Prat M, Yébenes JC. The Role of Water Homeostasis in Muscle Function and Frailty: A Review. Nutrients. 2019 Aug 9;11(8):1857. doi: 10.3390/nu11081857. PMID: 31405072; PMCID: PMC6723611.

Pross N. Effects of Dehydration on Brain Functioning: A Life-Span Perspective. Ann Nutr Metab. 2017;70 Suppl 1:30-36. doi: 10.1159/000463060. Epub 2017 Jun 15. PMID: 28614811.

Benton D. Dehydration influences mood and cognition: a plausible hypothesis? Nutrients. 2011 May;3(5):555-73. doi: 10.3390/nu3050555. Epub 2011 May 10. PMID: 22254111; PMCID: PMC3257694.

Kempton MJ, Ettinger U, Foster R, Williams SC, Calvert GA, Hampshire A, Zelaya FO, O'Gorman RL, McMorris T, Owen AM, Smith MS. Dehydration affects brain structure and function in healthy adolescents. Hum Brain Mapp. 2011 Jan;32(1):71-9. doi: 10.1002/hbm.20999. PMID: 20336685; PMCID: PMC6869970.

McMorris T, Swain J, Smith M, Corbett J, Delves S, Sale C, Harris RC, Potter J. Heat stress, plasma concentrations of adrenaline, noradrenaline, 5-hydroxytryptamine and cortisol, mood state and cognitive performance. Int J Psychophysiol. 2006 Aug;61(2):204-15. doi: 10.1016/j.ijpsycho.2005.10.002. Epub 2005 Nov 23. PMID: 16309771.

Hodges, Molly (2012) "The Effects of Dehydration on Cognitive Functioning, Mood, and Physical Performance,"The Corinthian: Vol. 13 , Article 2.Available at: https://kb.gcsu.edu/thecorinthian/vol13/iss1/2

Chapter 27

Wallace RK, et al. A wakeful hypometabolic physiologic state. American Journal of Physiology 221(3): 795-799, 1971

Schneider RH, et al. Stress Reduction in the Secondary Prevention of Cardiovascular Disease: Randomized, Controlled Trial of

Transcendental Meditation and Health Education in Blacks. Circ Cardiovasc Qual Outcomes 5:750-758, 2012

Travis FT and Shear J. Focused attention, open monitoring and automatic self-transcending: Categories to organize meditations from Vedic, Buddhist and Chinese traditions. Consciousness and Cognition 19(4):1110-1118, 2010

Rainforth MV, et al. Stress reduction programs in patients with elevated blood pressure: a systematic review and meta-analysis. Current Hypertension Reports 9:520–528, 2007

Brook RD, et al. Beyond Medications and Diet: Alternative Approaches to Lowering Blood Pressure. A Scientific Statement from the American Heart Association. Hypertension 61(6):1360-83, 2013

Cooper MJ, et al. Transcendental Meditation in the management of hypercholesterolemia. Journal of Human Stress 5(4): 24–27, 1979

Orme-Johnson DW and Walton KW. All approaches of preventing or reversing effects of stress are not the same. American Journal of Health Promotion 12:297-299, 1998

Barnes VA, et al. Impact of Transcendental Meditation on cardiovascular function at rest and during acute stress in adolescents with high normal blood pressure. Journal of Psychosomatic Research 51: 597-605, 2001

Jevning R, et al. Adrenocortical activity during meditation. Hormonal Behavior 10(1):54-60, 1978

Paul-Labrador M, et al. Effects of randomized controlled trial of Transcendental Meditation on components of the metabolic syndrome in subjects with coronary heart disease. Archives of Internal Medicine 166:1218-1224, 2006

Orme-Johnson DW, Herron RE. An Innovative Approach to Reducing Medical Care Utilization and Expenditures. American Journal of Managed Care 3: 135–144, 1997

Herron RE. Can the Transcendental Meditation Program Reduce the Medical Expenditures of Older People? A Longitudinal Cost-Reduction Study in Canada. Journal of Social Behavior and Personality 17(1): 415–442, 2005

Wallace RK, et al. The effects of the Transcendental Meditation and TM-Sidhi program on the aging process. International Journal of Neuroscience 16: 53-58, 1982

Glaser JL, Brind JL, Vogelman JH, Eisner MJ, Dillbeck MC, Wallace RK, Chopra D, Orentreich N. Elevated serum dehydroepiandrosterone sulfate levels in practitioners of the Transcendental Meditation (TM) and TM-Sidhi programs. J Behav Med. 1992 Aug;15(4):327-41. doi: 10.1007/BF00844726. PMID: 1404349.

Alexander CN, et al. Transcendental Meditation, mindfulness, and longevity. Journal of Personality and Social Psychology 57: 950-964, 1989

Alexander CN, et al. The effects of Transcendental Meditation compared to other methods of relaxation in reducing risk factors, morbidity, and mortality. Homeostasis 35: 243-264, 1994

Schneider RH, et al. Long-term effects of stress reduction on mortality in persons > 55 years of age with systemic hypertension. American Journal of Cardiology 95: 1060-1064, 2005

Duraimani S, et al. Effects of Lifestyle Modification on Telomerase Gene Expression in Hypertensive Patients: A Pilot Trial of Stress Reduction and Health Education Programs in African Americans. PLOS ONE 10(11): e0142689, 2015

Wenuganen S, Walton KG, Katta S, Dalgard CL, Sukumar G, Starr J, Travis FT, Wallace RK, Morehead P, Lonsdorf NK, Srivastava M, Fagan J. Transcriptomics of Long-Term Meditation Practice: Evidence for Prevention or Reversal of Stress Effects Harmful to Health. Medicina (Kaunas) 57(3): 218, 2021

Alexander CN, et al. Transcendental Meditation, self-actualization, and psychological health: A conceptual overview and statistical meta-analysis. Journal of Social Behavior and Personality 6: 189-247, 1991

Eppley KR, et al. Differential effects of relaxation techniques on trait anxiety: A meta-analysis. Journal of Clinical Psychology 45: 957-974, 1989

Alexander CN, et al. Effects of the Transcendental Meditation program on stress-reduction, health, and employee development: A prospective study in two occupational settings. Stress, Anxiety and Coping 6: 245–262, 1993

Harung HS, et al. Peak performance and higher states of consciousness: A study of world-class performers. Journal of Managerial Psychology 11(4): 3–23, 1996

Nidich S, et al. Non-trauma-focused meditation versus exposure therapy in veterans with post-traumatic stress disorder: a randomised controlled trial. Lancet Psychiatry 5(12):975-986, 2018

Wallace RK, Wallace T. Neuroadaptability and Habit: Modern Medicine and Ayurveda. Medicina (Kaunas). 2021 Jan 21;57(2):90. doi: 10.3390/medicina57020090. PMID: 33494269; PMCID: PMC7909780

Burke A, Lam CN, Stussman B, Yang H. Prevalence and patterns of use of mantra, mindfulness and spiritual meditation among adults in the United States. BMC Complement Altern Med. 2017 Jun 15;17(1):316. doi:

10.1186/s12906-017-1827-8. PMID: 28619092; PMCID: PMC5472955..

Chapter 28

Dfarhud D, Malmir M, Khanahmadi M. Happiness & Health: The Biological Factors- Systematic Review Article. Iran J Public Health. 2014 Nov;43(11):1468-77. PMID: 26060713; PMCID: PMC4449495.

Bakshi A, Tadi P. Biochemistry, Serotonin. 2022 Oct 5. In: StatPearls [Internet]. Treasure Island (FL): StatPearls Publishing; 2024 Jan–. PMID: 32809691.

Jones LA, Sun EW, Martin AM, Keating DJ. The ever-changing roles of serotonin. Int J Biochem Cell Biol. 2020 Aug;125:105776. doi: 10.1016/j.biocel.2020.105776. Epub 2020 May 29. PMID: 32479926.

Love TM. Oxytocin, motivation and the role of dopamine. Pharmacol Biochem Behav. 2014 Apr;119:49-60. doi: 10.1016/j.pbb.2013.06.011. Epub 2013 Jul 9. PMID: 23850525; PMCID: PMC3877159

Alexander R, Aragón OR, Bookwala J, Cherbuin N, Gatt JM, Kahrilas IJ, Kästner N, Lawrence A, Lowe L, Morrison RG, Mueller SC, Nusslock R, Papadelis C, Polnaszek KL, Helene Richter S, Silton RL, Styliadis C. The neuroscience of positive emotions and affect: Implications for cultivating happiness and wellbeing. Neurosci Biobehav Rev. 2021 Feb;121:220-249. doi: 10.1016/j.neubiorev.2020.12.002. Epub 2020 Dec

8. PMID: 33307046.

An HY, Chen W, Wang CW, Yang HF, Huang WT, Fan SY. The Relationships between Physical Activity and Life Satisfaction and Happiness among Young, Middle-Aged, and Older Adults. Int J Environ Res Public Health. 2020 Jul 4;17(13):4817. doi: 10.3390/ijerph17134817. PMID: 32635457; PMCID: PMC7369812.

Steptoe A, Deaton A, Stone AA. Subjective wellbeing, health, and ageing. Lancet. 2015 Feb 14;385(9968):640-648. doi: 10.1016/S0140-6736(13)61489-0. Epub 2014 Nov 6. PMID: 25468152; PMCID: PMC4339610.

Chapter 29

Caldwell HK, Albers HE. Oxytocin, Vasopressin, and the Motivational Forces that Drive Social Behaviors. Curr Top Behav Neurosci. 2016;27:51-103. doi: 10.1007/7854_2015_390. PMID: 26472550.

Froemke RC, Young LJ. Oxytocin, Neural Plasticity, and Social Behavior. Annu Rev Neurosci. 2021 Jul 8;44:359-381. doi: 10.1146/annurev-neuro-102320-102847. Epub 2021 Apr 6. PMID: 33823654; PMCID: PMC8604207.

Dharma Parenting: Understand Your Child's Brilliant Brain for Greater Happiness, Health, Success, and Fulfillment by Robert Keith Wallace, PhD, and Frederick Travis, PhD, Tarcher/Perigree, 2016

Chapter 30

Mohandas E. Neurobiology of spirituality. Mens Sana Monogr. 2008 Jan;6(1):63-80. doi: 10.4103/0973-1229.33001. PMID: 22013351; PMCID: PMC3190564.

Ramakrishnan P. 'You are here': locating 'spirituality' on the map of the current medical world. Curr Opin Psychiatry. 2015 Sep;28(5):393-401. doi: 10.1097/YCO.0000000000000180. PMID: 26164614.

Sherman R, Hickner J. Academic physicians use placebos in clinical practice and believe in the mind-body connection. J Gen Intern Med. 2008 Jan;23(1):7-10. doi: 10.1007/s11606-007-0332-z. Epub 2007 Nov 10. PMID: 17994270; PMCID: PMC2173915.

Ortega Á, Salazar J, Galban N, Rojas M, Ariza D, Chávez-Castillo M, Nava M, Riaño-Garzón ME, Díaz-CAmargo EA, Medina-Ortiz O, Bermúdez V. Psycho-Neuro-Endocrine-Immunological Basis of the Placebo Effect: Potential Applications beyond Pain Therapy. Int J Mol Sci. 2022 Apr 11;23(8):4196. doi: 10.3390/ijms23084196. PMID: 35457014; PMCID: PMC9028312.

Tavel M.E. The Placebo Effect: The Good, the Bad, and the Ugly. Am. J. Med. 2014;127:484–488. doi:10.1016/j.amjmed.2014.02.002.

Wager T.D., Atlas L.Y. The Neuroscience of Placebo Effects: Connecting Context, Learning and Health. Nat. Rev. Neurosci. 2015;16:403–418. doi: 10.1038/nrn3976

Bernstein MH, Brown WA. The placebo effect in psychiatric practice. Curr Psychiatr. 2017 Nov;16(11):29-34. PMID: 29910696; PMCID: PMC6003660.

Zion SR, Crum AJ. Mindsets Matter: A New Framework for Harnessing the Placebo Effect in Modern Medicine. Int Rev Neurobiol. 2018;138:137-160. doi: 10.1016/bs.irn.2018.02.002. Epub 2018 Mar 20. PMID: 29681322.

Crum AJ, Langer EJ. Mind-set matters: exercise and the placebo effect. Psychol Sci. 2007 Feb;18(2):165-71. doi: 10.1111/j.1467-9280.2007.01867.x. PMID: 17425538.

Human Physiology: Expression of Veda and the Vedic Literature 4th Edition by Dr. Tony Nader, MD, PhD, Maharishi Vedic University; 2001

Ramanyan in Human Physiology, by Dr. Tony Nader, MD, PhD, Maharishi Vedic University; 4th edition, 2001

One Unbounded Ocean of Consciousness: Simple Answers to Big Questions in Life by Dr. Tony Nader, MD, PhD, Penguin Random House Grupo Editorial, 2021

The Hero with a Thousand Faces by Joseph Campbell, New World Library; Third edition, 2008

Estebsari F, Dastoorpoor M, Khalifehkandi ZR, Nouri A, Mostafaei D, Hosseini M, Esmaeili R, Aghababaeian H. The Concept of Successful Aging: A Review Article. Curr Aging Sci. 2020;13(1):4-10. doi: 10.2174/1874609812666191023130117. PMID: 31657693; PMCID: PMC7403646.

Science of Being and Art of Living: Transcendental Meditation by Maharishi Mahesh Yogi, MUM Press, Kindle edition, 2011

Maharishi Mahesh Yogi on the Bhagavad-Gita, A New Translation and Commentary, Chapters 1-6, MUM Press, 2016

The Supreme Awakening: Experiences of Enlightenment Throughout Time –And How You Can Cultivate Them by Craig Pearson, MIU Press, 2013

Chapter 31

The Coherence Effect: Tapping into the Laws of Nature that Govern Health, Happiness, and Higher Brain Functioning by Robert Keith Wallace, PhD, Jay B. Marcus, and Chris S. Clark, MD, Armin Lear Press, 2020

The Neurophysiology of Enlightenment: How the Transcendental Meditation and TM-Sidhi Program Transform the Functioning of the Human Body by Robert Keith Wallace, PhD, Dharma Publications, 2016

Hagelin JS, et al. Effects of group practice of the Transcendental Meditation program on preventing violent crime in Washington, DC: results of the National Demonstration Project, June-July 1993. Social Indicators Research 47: 153-201, 1999

Orme-Johnson DW, et al. International peace project in the Middle East: The effect of the Maharishi Technology of the Unified Field. Journal of Conflict Resolution 32: 776–812, 1988

Orme-Johnson DW, et al. The long-term effects of the Maharishi Technology of the Unified Field on the quality of life in the United States (1960 to 1983). Social Science Perspectives Journal 2:127-146, 1988

Orme-Johnson DW, et al. Preventing terrorism and international conflict: Effects of large assemblies of participants in the Transcendental Meditation and TM-Sidhi programs. Journal of Offender Rehabilitation

36: 283–302, 2003

Brown CL. Overcoming barriers to use of promising research among elite Middle East policy groups. Journal of Social Behavior and Personality 17:489-546, 2005

Cavanaugh KL. Time series analysis of U.S. and Canadian inflation and unemployment: A test of a field-theoretic hypothesis. Proceedings of the American Statistical Association, Business and Economics Statistics Section (Alexandria, VA: American Statistical Association): 799–804, 1987

Cavanaugh KL, King KD. Simultaneous transfer function analysis of Okun's misery index: Improvements in the economic quality of life through Maharishi's Vedic Science and technology of consciousness. Proceedings of the American Statistical Association, Business and Economics Statistics Section (Alexandria, VA: American Statistical Association): 491–496, 1988

Davies JL. Alleviating political violence through enhancing coherence in collective consciousness. Dissertation Abstracts International 49(8): 2381A, 1989

Gelderloos P, et al. The dynamics of US–Soviet relations, 1979–1986: Effects of reducing social stress through the Transcendental Meditation and TM-Sidhi program. Proceedings of the Social Statistics Section of the American Statistical Association (Alexandria, VA: American Statistical Association): 297–302, 1990

Dillbeck MC. Test of a field theory of consciousness and social change: Time series analysis of participation in the TM-Sidhi program and reduction of violent death in the U.S. Social Indicators Research 22: 399–418, 1990

Assimakis PD, Dillbeck MC. Time series analysis of improved quality of life in Canada: Social change, collective consciousness, and the TM-Sidhi program. Psychological Reports 76: 1171–1193, 1995

Hatchard GD, et al. A model for social improvement. Time series analysis of a phase transition to reduced crime in Merseyside metropolitan area. Psychology, Crime, and Law 2: 165–174, 1996

Dillbeck MC, et al. The Transcendental Meditation program and crime rate change in a sample of forty-eight cities. Journal of Crime and

Justice 4: 25–45, 1981

Dillbeck MC, et al. Test of a field model of consciousness and social change: The Transcendental Meditation and TM-Sidhi program and decreased urban crime. The Journal of Mind and Behavior 9: 457–486, 1988

Dillbeck MC. et al. Consciousness as a field: The Transcendental Meditation and TM-Sidhi program and changes in social indicators. The Journal of Mind and Behavior 8: 67–104, 1987.

ABOUT THE AUTHORS

DR. ROBERT KEITH WALLACE

Robert Keith Wallace, PhD did pioneering research on the Transcendental Meditation technique. His seminal papers—published in *Science, American Journal of Physiology,* and *Scientific American*—on a fourth major state of consciousness support a new paradigm of mind-body medicine and total brain development. Dr. Wallace is the founding President of Maharishi International University, has traveled around the world giving lectures at major universities and institutes, and has written and co-authored many books.

He is presently a Trustee of Maharishi International University and Chairman of the Department of Physiology and Health.

TED WALLACE

Ted Wallace, MS is currently an Agile Coach at Principal Financial Group. He has completed two Master of Science degrees, one in Computer Science and the other in Physiology, at Maharishi International University. He is a certified Scrum Master Professional (CSM, CSPO, CSP, CTC) and a registered corporate coach (RCC) with thousands of hours of coaching sessions.

CAROL PAREDES

Carol Paredes, MS is the Associate Chair of the Department of Physiology & Health and Instructor of Physiology and Health. She is an integrative health coach, yoga teacher, and educator. She became a certified health coach after working more than 30 years in technology as a senior level engineer. Now she is responsible for managing the operations of the Department of Physiology and Health and assists in the development of the curriculum for the MS in Maharishi AyurVeda & Integrative Medicine and the MS in Aromatherapy and Ayurveda in addition to working on her PhD in Physiology and Health. Carol has a passion for helping clients, students, and staff integrate and benefit from the knowledge and practices of Maharishi AyurVeda.

ACKNOWLEDGMENTS

We would like to thank Allen Cobb for his ongoing help with Illustrator and InDesign.

INDEX

A

acetylcholine 16
addiction 14, 298
adrenaline 14
agni 67, 69, 70, 71
Alzheimer's 16, 301, 310
Ama 69, 153, 271
anticipation 18
anxiety 15, 68, 70, 309, 317, 322
aromatherapy 258, 319
ashwagandha 308
attention 281, 285
Ayurgenomics 265, 268
Ayurveda iv, 72, 128, 268, 269, 275, 278, 281, 285, 296, 305, 307, 312, 323

B

balance 257, 258, 259, 260, 261, 262, 263, 264, 265, 267
blood pressure 321
brahmi 309
brain wave 281
Breathwork 197

C

coherence 327
Cold Therapy viii
collective consciousness 289, 290, 292
consciousness iv, 247, 280, 286, 288, 289, 290, 292, 298, 299, 300, 301, 304,
    321, 325, 328
Curcumin 310

D

dementia 315
depression 15, 309, 316, 317
detoxification 70, 153, 312
digestion 257, 259, 260, 261, 262, 263, 264, 265
dopamine 14, 18, 19, 70, 72, 272, 274, 296, 298

E

endorphins 18
Energy State 257, 258, 259, 260, 261, 262, 264, 265
Energy States 76, 264
epigenetic 267
epilepsy 15
epinephrine 14
exercise 258, 259, 260, 262, 264, 265, 267, 268
experiment 130

F

fight or flight 14, 18

G

GABA 15, 70, 273
glutamate 16
gluten 274
gut-brain axis 153

H

habit 127, 128, 129, 130, 131
Habit Map 128, 129
Habit Plan 130
happiness 15, 265, 288, 323
health 261, 264, 281, 282, 283, 284, 287, 288
"Here-and-Now" neurotransmitters 18, 19
higher states of consciousness 323
hydration 205

I

impulse control 15

K

Kapha 128, 129, 265, 266, 267, 278, 279
K Energy State 76

L

learning 14, 16, 72

longevity 153, 280, 322
L-theanine 314

M

magnesium 314
Maharishi ii, iv, v, 70, 71, 280, 298, 299, 300, 301, 304, 312, 325, 326, 327, 329
Maharishi Ayurveda v, 70, 71, 312
Maharishi Mahesh Yogi 289
Maharishi Mahesh Yogi, 289
meditation v, 71, 213, 281, 282, 285, 286, 287, 288, 295, 296, 298, 317, 321,
        322, 323, 326, 327, 328, 329
melatonin 302, 303, 313, 314
memory 16, 296
microbiome 267
mitochondria 302, 313
motivation 14, 19, 265, 274, 288
movement 14, 68

N

nervous system 281, 282
neurons 15, 16
Neuroscience 287
neurotransmitter 13, 15, 70, 71
noradrenaline 14
norepinephrine 14, 18

O

Ojas 119
Omega-3s 311
oxytocin 18

P

panchakarma 70, 153
Paul 286
P Energy State 75, 128, 131, 258, 259, 261, 262, 265
performance 265, 288
personalize 72
Pitta 128, 129, 265, 266, 267, 277
PK Energy State 262
Prakriti 265, 268, 269

prebiotics 153
prefrontal cortex 299
probiotics 153

R

relationships 263
Rest and Repair Diet 265, 288

S

Selye 295
serotonin 15, 18
sleep 15, 75, 258, 259, 264, 265, 313, 314, 315, 317
Soma 119
spirituality 239
stress 15, 69, 70, 71, 74, 75, 76, 273, 295, 296, 309, 310, 321, 322, 323, 327
sugar 276
sunlight 300, 303
suprachiasmatic nucleus 300

T

therapy 288
TM v, 281, 282, 283, 284, 285, 287, 289, 290, 291, 292, 293, 295, 319, 322, 326, 327, 328
toxins 67, 69, 70, 272
Transcendental Meditation v, 281, 282, 283, 284, 286, 287, 288, 289, 291, 292, 293, 295, 296, 298, 321, 322, 326, 327, 328, 329
triphala 307
turmeric 278, 280

V

Vata 265, 266, 267, 274, 275
V Energy State 74, 257, 258, 261, 262, 265
Vitamin D 311
VK Energy State 262
VP Energy State 260, 261
VPK Energy State 264

Y

yoga 258

Index

www.ingramcontent.com/pod-product-compliance
Lightning Source LLC
Chambersburg PA
CBHW031116020426
42333CB00012B/108